Fifteen Steps Out of Darkness

Fifteen Steps Out of Darkness

The Way of the Cross for People on the Journey of Mental Illness

By Scott Rose, Fred Wenner, and Al Rose
Artwork by Homer Yost
Prologue by Therese Borchard

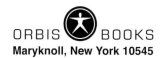
ORBIS BOOKS
Maryknoll, New York 10545

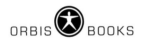 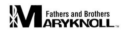

Founded in 1970, Orbis Books endeavors to publish works that enlighten the mind, nourish the spirit, and challenge the conscience. The publishing arm of the Maryknoll Fathers and Brothers, Orbis seeks to explore the global dimensions of the Christian faith and mission, to invite dialogue with diverse cultures and religious traditions, and to serve the cause of reconciliation and peace. The books published reflect the views of their authors and do not represent the official position of the Maryknoll Society. To learn more about Maryknoll and Orbis Books, please visit our website at www.maryknollsociety.org.

Library of Congress Cataloging-in-Publication Data

Rose, Scott (CEO)
    Fifteen steps out of darkness : the way of the cross for people on the journey of
    mental illness / by Scott Rose, Fred Wenner, and Al Rose ; artwork by Homer Yost ;
    prologue by Therese Borchard.
        pages cm
    ISBN 978-1-62698-182-9 (pbk.)
    1. Stations of the Cross--Meditations 2. Mentally ill—Religious life. 3. De
    pressed persons—Religious life. I. Title.
    BX2040.R67 2016
                            232.96—dc23

For
Fred and Walter Barbe

With Gratitude to
The Foundation for Spirituality and Medicine

The people who walked in darkness have seen a great light.

—Isaiah 9:1

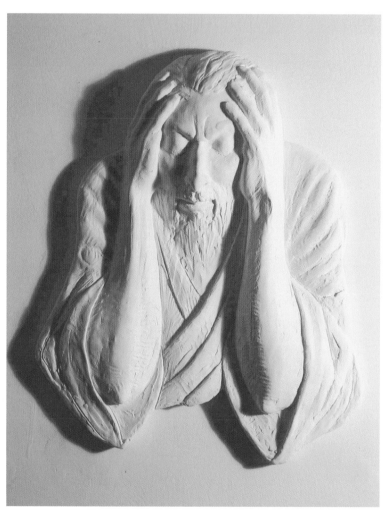

Gethsemane

CONTENTS

Contents

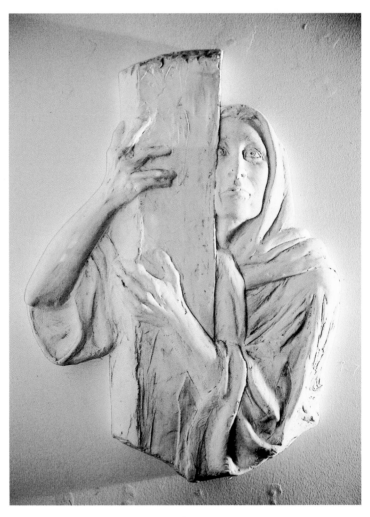

Mary at the Cross

PROLOGUE

Therese Borchard

I can still smell the incense from those Friday afternoons during Lent at St. Charles Borromeo Grade School where the entire school crowded in the modern chapel to celebrate the Stations of the Cross. Approximately eight hundred kids would begin each station by singing, "Were You There (When They Crucified My Lord)?" Then a narrator would name the station and briefly described what happened. A second narrator would read a reflection that tried to relate the station to our lives. There was a slide show to accompany each narrator. One picture of Jesus falling or meeting the women (or another station), and one image of a modern-day problem: often photos of hungry people in Africa and victims of child abuse.

I remember wishing on those afternoons that I were starving so that my pain would be legitimate, so that I could associate the aching hole inside of me with the blood of Jesus as he was crucified. The images on the slides were acknowledged forms of suffering. If you had to fill out a form to qualify for valid reasons to hurt, you could definitely place a checkmark next to "starving to death" or "victim of child abuse." Whatever was going on inside my head as a young girl, though, failed that qualification.

So I suffered in silence. Alone. I didn't tell anyone that I wanted to die. That is why this book is so important.

The slideshow tells of a different kind of suffering from all the slideshows in grade schools around the world. For the very first time, the Stations of the Cross are told from the perspective of those living with serious mental illness and those who support them as family, mental health professionals, and volunteer caregivers. The anguish that I sat with silently as a young girl is finally acknowledged and put in the context of the greatest Christian story: the death and resurrection of Jesus. It's as if the authors have said to me and have said to everyone who is affected by my mental illness (my husband, my psychiatrist, my therapist, my friends), "Yes, you were right to look to the Cross for hope."

"It is so hard to heal from mental illness," Way Station CEO Scott Rose, one of the authors of this book, said to me the day I visited Way Station's Psychiatric Rehabilitation Program, "There is no cure yet for this brain disease."

Way Station is an organization that provides mental health care, housing, and employment services to over three thousand low-income adults and children in Maryland with severe mental illness as well as developmental disabilities and substance addictions. The huge-hearted people who work there embrace principles of resilience and recovery—teaching individuals how to live with their conditions or manage their symptoms, as opposed to expecting a cure or closing their eyes and wishing it would all just disappear. The process of recovery is a life-long journey.

Clearly everyone around the person with the illness is also challenged by it. Family members and caregivers are often overwhelmed with the emotions surrounding mental illness, challenged by the despair, and angry when trying to help people is so unsuccessful. The healing process for *all* affected involves learning to cope.

Not unlike the experiences of all three authors, my husband once explained to me how difficult it was for him to watch the woman he loves suffer so intensely. I noticed extra creases form around his eyes and a fatigue in the way he held his shoulders. There was a feeling of helplessness and urgency, a frustrating lack of control.

Fred Wenner, one of the authors, is a retired Protestant minister who parented fifty-three foster children with his wife, many of whom had emotional challenges.

They adopted four, adding them to their family of four biological children. Three of their adopted and foster children were served by Way Station. After a career as a university professor of literature, Al Rose, another author, worked as a chaplain at a maximum security prison, then as a chaplain of an inner-city hospice, and later as a volunteer for Way Station. The artwork was created by Homer Yost, a professional sculptor with bipolar disorder who was served by Way Station when the organization was formed in the early 1980s.

This book will resonate with caregivers and family members as well as with people directly struggling with the illness like me. There are so many of us who are impacted by mental illness, either directly or indirectly. One out of every four adults suffers from a diagnosable mental illness in any given year. One out of every sixteen individuals has a more severe form of mental illness such as schizophrenia or bipolar disorder from which I suffer. One out of every four families has a loved one with a severe mental illness. And there are about 2.4 million people working in the mental health field.

I recognized my struggles in the individuals I met at Way Station with severe mental illness, some of whom appear in the following chapters (for the most part, names have been changed for privacy). I related to the gentleman who was trying to keep his job despite hearing loud voices. My voices are different. They are "death thoughts"—obsessions about getting to the other side and being able to rest with Jesus—but they distract me as if they were the voices he talks about. And yes, it can be very difficult for me to concentrate and do my job. I also felt for the young guy who was trying to come back to his faith after a painful bout of scrupulosity and obsessive-compulsive disorder. For me the line is tenuous between ardent piety and disease symptoms.

Viktor E. Frankl, M.D., Ph.D., holocaust survivor, and author of "Man's Search for Meaning," once said that "everyone has his or her Auschwitz," that one can never compare suffering. However, my trip to Way Station was humbling because I knew that after my visit, I would return to a loving family, a home in an okay part of town, and a healthy, cooked meal. Few of the individuals there could say that. I was among the lucky ones, as a mother, wife, and writer.

I was truly humbled by the courage and perseverance on display there, the same persistence and determination that is captured in the narratives included in this book. These people live complex, messy lives. They fall and fall again. Their flesh is punctured. They are stripped of their pride. And just when you think someone has approached the resurrection chapter, that person begins to stumble. True to life, the experiences of resurrection in this book are followed by setbacks.

But that's where the hope is.

The Prophet Isaiah speaks of Jesus's coming when he says to the long-suffering Israelites, *The people who walked in darkness have seen a great light.* It is noteworthy that the Hebrew word for light is *or*, which means order, because the ancient Israelites believed that light brought order to the chaos of darkness and that God brought order to the disorder of misfortune. So it is with the physical and spiritual journey of recovery with mental illness: the goal is often to help people *manage* the symptoms rather than eliminating them—in the same way that light can help us manage darkness as opposed to dispelling it.

Jesus's walk to Calvary brings order to disorder and healing to disease. Although no resurrection lasts forever while we live here in this world, the Stations do provide fifteen profound steps out of darkness, and into hope, especially in the life-long journey of recovery with mental illness.

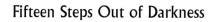

Fifteen Steps Out of Darkness

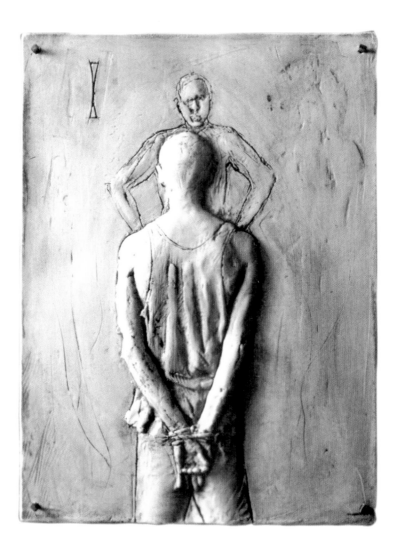

JESUS IS CONDEMNED

Scott Rose

The late anarchist Emma Goldman once said that it requires less mental effort to condemn than to think.

I guess Tom was smarter than anyone thought.

Over fifteen years ago, in one of the four Maryland counties Way Station has locations, we opened a house for individuals with mental illness. Some neighbors protested the move because they feared that our residents would cause physical harm to them and that their property values would go down. In particular, they feared that our ragged, middle-aged men would assault the females of the neighborhood.

Our residents were clearly the bad guys. Maybe the neighbors didn't fault them for having a disability, but the judgments were heard loud and clear. Our folks malingered on welfare under the subterfuge of mental illness. They lacked the resolve to take their medication. They weren't strong enough to stop their addictions to alcohol or drugs.

Big Tom, a three-hundred-pound, six-foot tall, middle-aged resident of that house? He seemed to represent all that those neighbors feared. The neighbors felt that the way to keep their neighborhood safe and prosperous was to have fewer people with mental illness and more police officers to address a recent increase in crime (which, by the way, was not due to our residents). Because the Federal Fair Housing Act was amended in 1988 to add people with disabilities as a protected class with regard to housing discrimination, neighbors knew that they could not prevent our residents from living there. But pressure mounted to convince us to relocate. As much as we tried to insulate Tom and the other residents from this prejudice, they knew they were not welcome.

What's worse: the pain of mental illness or the injustice of the discrimination toward people who suffer from the disease? I've often wondered that when I speak to caregivers, family members, or professionals. Like most people, I grieve when someone I care about experiences the haunting loneliness of depression or the terror of fear and paranoia. But when that vulnerable client or loved one is being treated unkindly? There is a frustration that wells up inside—on top of the grief—and sometimes guilt on top of both of those, because I am not able to protect the individual. I feel inadequate and powerless. I can only imagine how much harder it is for families—and for the individuals.

The story that the neighbors expected took an unexpected turn. One night, the adult relative of elderly neighbors pounded on the door of the house, screaming that her husband was going to shoot her and pleading to be let it. Without thinking, Tom opened the door. His impulsiveness—which was his greatest weakness—drove him toward making the loving choice, despite its risk. The woman rushed in, and a man with a gun came right behind her. Tom wrestled with the man, pushed him out the door, and locked it. Having intended to commit a domestic murder–suicide, the man ended the violence on the lawn of our house by shooting himself in the head. The next day, it became clear that the husband was an off-duty police officer, exactly the kind of person the neighbors wanted more of.

I was incredibly proud of Tom for his act of bravery. But I was astounded that the hero who saved a neighbor from her death did not receive one gesture of thanks. Had Tom not been wearing the label *Way Station client*, had the protesting neighbors not already made their minds up that he was costing them thousands of dollars each year in property values, then he would have been the recipient of homemade apple pies, caramel cakes, and cards. Some may have shed tears of gratitude.

What was even more surprising, though, was that Tom didn't expect any kind of appreciation. Staff and clients applauded his heroism, but he received it with embarrassment and was truly perplexed, as it just seemed to him that any person, with or without a disability, would have done the same.

Neither response seemed right to me. So I vowed to tell the whole story. I believed that when the neighbors and the rest of the area heard all the facts, they would have a different view of Tom and might even recognize him to be the hero that he was. I wanted to use his story to teach a great lesson about the goodness and courage of people with mental illness. I had no desire to vilify the officer—I just wanted to explain how much more of a hero Tom was. We had then, and still do have, a wonderful collaboration with law enforcement in all Maryland jurisdictions in which Way Station has locations. But surely a lesson was due here, and the facts that exposed the contrast between Tom and the officer were essential to that lesson.

However, by the middle of the next day, it became clear that the public was not likely to learn about Tom's heroism. The media release only noted that the officer had committed suicide. No mention was made about the prior events or that he had tried to shoot his wife. Knowing that the reporter would be getting to me by that evening for a follow-up story, I began to prepare my response. I wanted so badly to tell the whole truth—whether I was asked or not. I believed that the officer, unfortunately, needed to be condemned so that the Way Station residents could be freed, released from this unfair prejudice that had shackled them for so much of their lives.

I prayed for guidance, and it came. All of a sudden, I realized that the officer was one of us. And that the neighbors were us, too. The officer obviously had mental illness—he committed suicide, after all. And the wife was suffering from trauma, her relatives from fear and anxiety for their loved one. The other neighbors who opposed us were reacting out of misguided fears. My righteous indignation with the neighborhood discrimination was so powerful that it blinded me from recognizing a suicide victim as a fellow traveler on the journey of mental illness. The officer was the suffering Christ whom I was about to condemn, in the same way that the neighbors condemned our residents.

I chose to keep the rest of the real truth in my heart at that time and for the near future. The reporter never asked, and I didn't offer. Only a decade later can I now share the full story, with the passing of time and the buffer of anonymity.

It is completely understandable that individuals with mental illness, their families, and caregivers get frustrated and angry with the various forms of injustice that surround mental illness. The arbitrariness of who gets the disease, the elusiveness of a cure, the unfairness of discrimination. We are hit by so many wrongs that we sometimes think we, in turn, need to condemn someone else to make things right. But the pain doesn't lessen if we further blame. We just get angrier. And we end up pushing another body into the dirt road of suffering on which Jesus carried his cross.

Mental illness is an injustice that, like any other ailment or condition, is difficult to comprehend, let alone to accept. Many people with mental illness, family members, and caregivers, are like Tom, with no hero report in hand. The valiant efforts they make in our communities—not to mention in their own minds, defeating thought after thought—will rarely be written up as braveness. And yet, if we try following Jesus to Calvary, starting with this first station, we may lose our anger to love, our sadness to hope, and our guilt to redemption.

In the first station, Jesus gives himself to us in vulnerability, allowing himself to be condemned. With this act of humility, he permits the story of his death and resurrection to begin. Tom, also, was vulnerable in his mental illness. His disease, with its oftentimes dysfunctional impulsiveness and naivety, allowed him to save a woman from her death, to redeem her husband, and to inspire me with humility and insight as to why the story of the cross begins with condemnation.

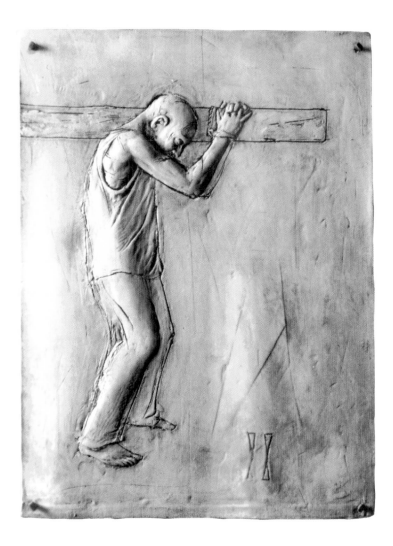

JESUS CARRIES HIS CROSS
Al Rose

Cal was a small man with wispy blonde hair going grey, round face raggedly shaved, who shuffled and spoke with some difficulty. His severe mental disability prevented him from participating in conversations, which often he couldn't follow. He could, however, occasionally express an idea in a relatively coherent way. I saw him in the building and we would exchange hellos, but we never came into closer contact, quite honestly because talking with him was so difficult. If I approached to chat, he would look at me blankly and then break into a smile and recount something about a relative, quite unconnected with the question I had asked.

Then a friend called me from my parish. It seemed that Cal was a Catholic, and my friend was a Eucharistic minister who brought communion to him weekly, at Cal's assisted living facility. In the course of talking to Cal, my friend discovered that Cal came to the program where I volunteered and knew who I was. My friend was going on vacation and wondered if I could substitute for him, bringing communion to Cal, while my friend was gone. I said of course.

After parking on a street in a decaying area of the city, I found it: a dingy clapboard house in an old, shabby neighborhood. Up the unpainted steps was an unpainted ramp for the disabled. I rang and was ushered into a front sitting room, cluttered with worn furniture and crowded with the folks living there. In some ways, it reminded me a bit of the houses I had gone into while a home-care chaplain in the inner city. I walked into the dining room where more residents sat around the table, some talking, others in chairs around the room, sitting alone, unspeaking, with their thoughts or with their pain. I found Cal there. No privacy, but we talked quietly at a corner of the table.

I learned Cal's sad story, in pieces, over several visits. He had been raised in a Catholic parish, but he had been refused admission to the local Catholic high school because of his emotional and intellectual limitations. Clearly, the school had not had the capacity to deal with such a youngster. He told me this sadly, obviously hurt. Limited in so many ways as he might be, he clearly felt that in this instance, which at the time had been extremely important to him, he had been rejected by his church. His friends had gone on but he had had to stay behind, to go to special education in the public system.

But Cal had a sweet temperament, and, amazingly, he did not blame the Church. His hurt seemed simple, almost pure, uncomplicated by resentments of the people involved. I think that at first I expected anger toward the principal, or whoever had made the decision, and also perhaps toward a teacher, or whoever might have explained that he was being refused admission, even perhaps his pastor. Many people—most, I think—would have directed anger at someone for the decision. Or even at the messenger, whoever conveyed the sad news. I have hoped that the person who did tell him was kind, understanding. Cal simply never expressed anger toward anyone. He simply did not blame. He carried his pain without it. How like Jesus. Despite this rejection, this gentle little man had not wavered in his faith or in his loyalty to the church.

I covered for my friend several times after that, visiting Cal every week. I saw and felt such beauty in him. I would start the little rite from the Ordinary Rite of Communion for the Sick by saying, "The Lord be with you."

And Cal would respond, "And with you."

I would continue, "Lord have Mercy."

And he would repeat it without prompting as well as repeating, "Christ have mercy . . . Lord have mercy."

Somewhere, from someone, he had learned to respond this way. The first time, I was so surprised that afterward I asked where he had learned this. He had gone to his parish's elementary school, where those blessed sisters had stayed with him and done their best to help him along. (I know so many folks with a Catholic school background whose principal memory was of rulers swatted on their knuckles, including my own brother. But from Cal's sweet story, let's remember that wasn't a universal experience!)

Then I would read a small scripture passage, as called for in the rite. I tended to use the passages provided in that Ordinary Rite of Communion of the Sick. For instance, from John 14:23, "Jesus answered: 'Anyone who loves me will be true to my word, and my Father will love him; and we will make our dwelling place with him.'" Or from 1 John 4:16, "We have come to know and believe in the love God has for us. God is love, and he who lives in love, lives in God, and God in him." (I would change the text's "abide" into "live" in order to avoid a word not common in our spoken language any more. I think that the translator would have forgiven me!) I used just these two passages over and over. Repetitive yes, but they conveyed a simple, but profound, message that God loves us. I would say to him, "Cal, this says that God loves you and me. Isn't that wonderful?"

He would smile, nod, and say yes. Then we'd talk, as best we could, about God's love for us. Limited as Cal was, he quite clearly understood the concept of God's love.

That seems so right to me, as I think about Cal in relation to Jesus and his cross. It is all about love.

Then we would say the Our Father, which he could do in part on his own, in part repeating after me. It was the same with the response to "Lamb of God." Then we would take communion together.

When Jesus says we should be like children, he means in our trust of God. In Cal it was truly child-like, simple, devout, trusting, grateful. Ministering to him felt holy. And afterward, when we saw each other, I felt that we related to one another as people who had shared something very meaningful together—for me something quite precious.

Cal was an unassuming witness of God's pure love in my life. He was not rejected because he was hated or feared. No one shouting out "Barabbas." His rejection was more like Jesus's when he returned to Nazareth, in the sense that it was not violent, but rather a matter of not believing in his power. Cal was barred admission to Catholic high school because of an unthreatening lack of ability. And yet he has a beautiful spirit; a gentle, loving nature; a power that was, unfortunately, not sufficient in school. Many folks with mental illness, like Cal, embody that irony, in lacking a power recognized as necessary in society, and yet they are infused with the greater power of a loving soul.

Because of the humble and loving way with which Cal accepted God's will, in him I saw Jesus in his passion. It was the second station of the cross, right before me.

Jesus accepted his cross.

THIRD STATION

Jesus Falls the First Time
Fred Wenner

When Jesus fell the first time, or any time on his way to the crucifixion, I've often wondered about Joseph. Even if he had died several years earlier and may not have been there physically, he most certainly continued to be a strong spiritual presence in the life of his son. So, I wonder what is going on with Joseph, Jesus's *foster father*? Preceding the steps to Calvary, did he wake in the middle of the night in a sweat, followed by a surprising calm, like I did the second night on my Ignatian retreat? Was Joseph warned or consoled by a visiting angel at some point before his son's arrest?

Matthew and his twin brother, Wayne, came to us as foster babies in March of 1984. From the outset, the expectation of our foster care workers was that this would be a temporary placement in the hope that either

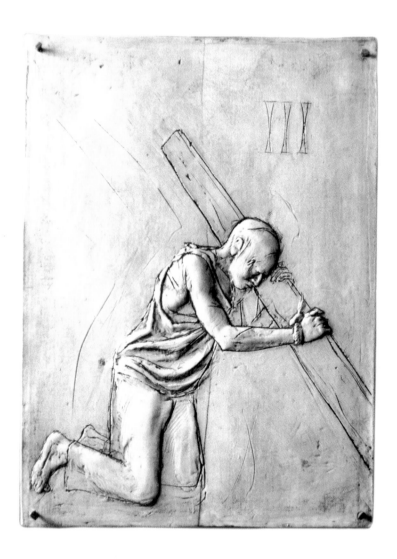

their biological parents would eventually be able to raise them or, failing that optimal scenario, the twins would be adopted by a loving family.

Two years later in the spring of 1986, Matt and Wayne were still with us, and the questions about their future had not been resolved when I left home for an eight-day religious retreat to get my head and heart together. Following the *Spiritual Exercises* of Ignatius of Loyola at a former Jesuit novitiate, I maintained a discipline of silence, broken only by the celebration of the Mass and a daily hour of teaching and debriefing with my spiritual director. It was a time of total immersion in God's word, when I was so prayerfully focused on scripture and my interior life that I actually entered the biblical stories and had enlightening conversations with the likes of Peter, Mary, and even Jesus. This discipline led me into an intense struggle with my faith, my vocation, my commitments, and the cost and joy of discipleship.

Although I had chosen a retreat setting for my getaway from the relentless press and stress of parish duties and family responsibilities, early on I discovered that I could not fully put aside my anxiety over *at home* issues in order to work on my spiritual issues. Foremost among these *distractions* (as viewed from the perspective of my spiritual director) was the fact that the twins were still with us, and it was very unclear as to what could be expected in terms of a plan for permanency in a family setting.

All of this came to a head during my second night on retreat when I awoke suddenly at 3 a.m. with something akin to an anxiety attack. Quite unexpectedly, my mind was in anguish over the fate of our foster sons. Since I left home, I had not been dwelling on the decisions that would soon have to be made for the twins, so I was surprised to find this issue front and center in the middle of the night. Actually, I was taken aback just by being awakened in such a state, because I am usually a very sound sleeper and I'm not used to spending my nights worrying about anything.

In my agitated state that night, I had a powerful sense of decisions being made for the twins, and I had no idea what those decisions might entail. My greatest fear was that I would discover when I got home that another family would be adopting the twins. I was in such a frenzy that I imagined being in a courtroom arguing against removing the boys from our family, and I was madly scribbling notes to make my case. I didn't sleep the rest of the night because my worries continued unabated, triggering a nasty headache and stomach cramps. Prayer was futile.

When morning light dawned, I finally got up, showered, and got dressed. Still, the issue of Matt and Wayne weighed heavily on my mind two days into my retreat, effectively blocking any fruitful or fulfilling prayer. But when I met with my spiritual director the next morning and talked through the strange experience of the previous night, my anxiety about my wife, Fran, and the twins' well-being began to ease. Eventually I discovered that I had no real worries whatsoever. There was growing in me a surprisingly sublime assurance that Fran and the family were safely in God's hands, as was I, and that was all I needed to know. So I was able to move on through the retreat, which led me deeper and became more fulfilling.

When I got home from the retreat, my anxiety attack began to make sense. I found out that a week before, on the very day when I awoke in such anguish, Fran received word that the twins would be freed for *open adoption*—which effectively means that what I was sensing was *good* news, not bad news. My anxiety was not well founded, but somehow I *knew* that something very significant was happening that very day. What on earth was going on? I can only conclude that it was not simply my imagination running wild; rather, it may have been a divine intrusion or a purposeful premonition (a visitation?) of some sort. My spiritual director dubbed it simply *a gift*.

Now, let me say a bit more about my son, Matt. When Matthew was born twelve weeks early, he weighed just over two pounds. His twin brother, born first, was a half-pound heavier, and it was clear from the outset that both of the boys would have some striking difficulties as they grew. Not only were they underweight and underdeveloped preemies, but their biological mother had been drinking heavily throughout her pregnancy, and she had no prenatal care.

When the twins were over four pounds each, because it was clear that their biological parents were not able and/or willing to care for them at that time, Matt and Wayne were released to our care and became our foster children. Throughout their first year, the boys were hooked up to electronic monitors to alert us if their heart beats or their breathing became irregular or stopped. Needless to say, we had a few scares. Then, when the twins were two-and-one-half years old, they were adopted into the Wenner family.

Actually, one could say that Matthew and Wayne were wired from the start. Apart from having electrodes all over their little bodies, after they outgrew their need for the monitors, they were diagnosed with Attention Deficit Disorder, exacerbated by having the residual effects of Fetal Alcohol Syndrome. As they continued to grow, serious learning disabilities became evident; and as they reached adolescence, both have had to battle depression and a nasty addiction to alcohol and other drugs. Eventually Matt was diagnosed with bipolar disorder, and he's now struggling with schizoaffective disorder as well.

While formal education was challenging for both of the boys because of their learning disabilities, Wayne was able to go on to gainful, long-term employment. Matt, on the other hand, was unable to hold jobs for any period of time. When Matt was in his early twenties, he became a member of Way Station. In his first few years there, Matt entered the Dual Recovery Program. I was never so proud of him as the day he graduated. He's been able to remember the lessons he was taught in that program in order to manage a very fragile life that could easily take a wrong turn at any time.

It's fair to say that Matt's been something of an unlucky kid. Like Jesus on his way to the cross, he has fallen many times. Unjustly so. His problems since birth have been more serious than his twin brother's. He's very bright, but this quality is often hidden behind his more apparent mental illnesses. Matt's funny, too, but not always when he wants to be—like when he was walking home from school and his pants wound up around his ankles because he refused to wear a belt. He fell that day.

He also collapsed to the ground like Jesus the day he was hit by a car, tossed onto the car's hood and windshield, thrown onto the asphalt and then flown to a shock trauma unit in Baltimore. A couple years later, Matt made a bad mistake in letting an under-the-influence friend drive his car recklessly, crashing it and rolling it over. Matt came out of both accidents with no serious or long-lasting injuries, but he's been stitched up after family scuffles, and in one twelve-month period, he broke his glasses in eight separate incidents, ranging from crushing them under text books in his backpack to losing them in a neighbor's yard until a mower found them.

Fran and I have had numerous tiffs when one of us sees Matt's behavior caused by his mental illness, and the other sees it either as very intentional or just a normal part of his growing up. With children who have no discernable mental illness, the answer is relatively simple—this is just the way kids are and this is what kids do. With Matt, it's not so clear. He can be blamed for things over which he has little control, or he can be excused and evade responsibility for something he could, and should, control.

This can be tough for families, because it's excruciating for us to see our kids struggle, and it's likely that each family member of a person with mental illness may have a different understanding of the effects of such illnesses on a person's behavior. Consequently, there are bound to be family disagreements because of our differing perspectives: Is all this unavoidable . . . or intentional . . . or accidental . . . or shameful . . . or pitiful . . . or providential . . . or what? Parents spend lifetimes trying to sort this out. Sometimes we're right,

and sometimes we're wrong. Either way, there are consequences.

In my times of confusion and in my efforts to do
the right thing, I can often relate to the strange tale of
Joseph, the *foster father* of Jesus, whom I have learned to
know as *the befuddled one.* He stands aside as the angel
Gabriel makes a dramatic appearance to Mary to announce that she will become the mother of the world's
savior; and in her beautiful humility, she utters a song
of praise unparalleled in Christian literature. Out of the
limelight, Joseph watches this drama unfold with nothing to say but "huh?"

The gospel stories say that Joseph was visited by an
angel, too. However, it was a no-name angel that came
to him to tell him what was going on. And while the
visit of Gabriel to Mary is beautifully depicted in centu-
ries of Christian art and prose, I don't see much attention being paid to Joseph's visit by the angel when he
was feeling sidelined and needing to be assured that he
really was an important figure in his family's unfolding
drama. Oh yes, the angel of the Lord appeared to Joseph
in a dream . . . at night.

I'm still awed by that 3 a.m. experience during my
spiritual retreat, trying to make some sense of it twenty-
five years later. With Joseph's companionship, I may be
closer to some sense of resolution. I know that the experience really did point me toward an answer to our

prayers—we wanted to adopt Matt and Wayne, and it wasn't long until we did.

It must be terrifying to fall in the way that Jesus did and Matt does so often. However, I suspect it is just as terrifying to watch a fall from the perspective of a father. Visitations can be disturbing as well, at least initially. If that's what I experienced long ago, it probably ran true to form. However, I've also learned from the angel's visit to Joseph that, even though it must have been upsetting at first, eventually the angel's presence and message brought reassurance and a sense of peace with Joseph's very odd circumstances. My guess is that God must have provided Joseph—wherever he was—the same kind of assurance and hope during his son's bloodiest hours, carrying his cross to his death, just as he has done for me as I watch my son trudge along the wearisome road of mental illness, stumbling every so often.

Jesus Meets His Mother

Fred Wenner

"There is no coming to consciousness without pain," wrote Carl Jung. "People will do anything no matter how absurd, in order to avoid facing their own soul. One does not become enlightened by imagining figures of light, but by making the darkness conscious."

As a parent of a mentally ill child, you live in a state of constant consciousness. It is demanding, exasperating, and often exhausting. We simply can't do it without being grounded in the immense love of a gracious God, the same God who loves *all children,* especially those who wrestle so intensely with dark forces from within—those that can't, for whatever reason, face their own soul—and can't seem to access all the loving that we take for granted.

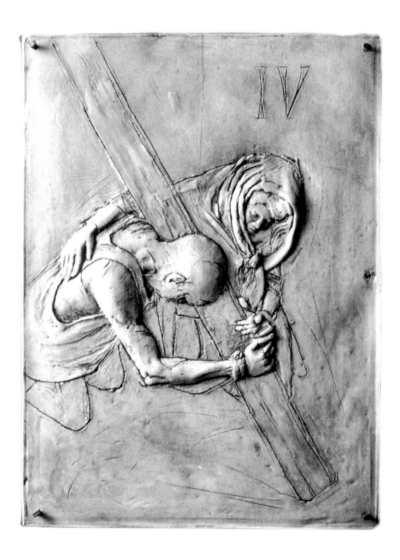

Melissa, our foster daughter, was one such child. She first arrived in 1980, when she was nine years old, and stayed with us for long stretches in the early '80s and then very sporadically in the late '80s. She was timid, apprehensive, always peering up at us from under of dense crop of light, frizzy hair.

Thirty years ago, foster parents were given very little information on the backgrounds of children, and our recollection is that Melissa said very little about her biological family, except that she occasionally spoke of her affection for her brothers. Her father was an alcoholic. I knew him as a regular guest at our homeless shelter in the early 1990s until he died when he fell down a flight of steps when he was drunk. Melissa's mother died of a heart attack in 1998. It's likely that Melissa either ran away from home or was taken from her home by court order—we're quite sure that she was designated a CINS (a child in need of supervision). Many of our teenage foster children were in that category.

We could see that she was deeply troubled, but we didn't have a name or diagnosis for her mental illness. She just was without that spark in her eye, the evidence of some passion tucked away inside to make her tick. She never seemed to be the beautiful child she must once have been. Melissa had a high-pitched, baby-sounding voice that always threw us off as to how old she really was. She sounded, and at times acted, as if she was almost an infant. We saw it as a cry for attention, but we could rarely do so to her satisfaction. She was prone to exaggeration, and we never knew what stories to believe. She enjoyed drama. For example, one morning she came down to breakfast wearing the prized jeans of her foster sister. It caused an immediate uproar when the sister loudly accused Melissa of stealing her jeans. I can still see that self-satisfied smirk on Melissa's face— that morning she got the attention she craved.

At one point, she left us with the hope of reuniting with her mother. Another time or two, she left our home to be adopted, but sadly it fell through. We also know that she was institutionalized during the late '80s—in a rehab center and in a group home for troubled girls.

She would leave for a while for one reason or another, and then she would be back with us. But before long, she'd be gone again. For weeks or years, we didn't know where she was or what she was up to. One time we heard that she was in Utah. She thought she had a computer chip in her. It's not uncommon for those dealing with paranoia to have unwarranted fears of somebody tracking them or controlling them, a fear that erodes their trust in just about everyone. Despite her fears, she hoped to study at a university, but she ended up homeless. Although her situations varied, there was always a profound sense of tragedy, a dark and ominous cloud, hovering over our dear Melissa.

We hadn't seen her for years when she called me at home and wanted to meet. I promised to meet her at my office at the church. The moment my eyes met hers that day I knew that my daughter felt she had some important spiritual work to do. She was wearing her past like a heavy, cumbersome coat that she was finally, after years of being constricted and weighed down, ready to shed. She clutched it tightly as a security item because it was all that she knew. And yet, tasting a sense of the freedom that might come from her confession, she faced her soul, and she confided in me.

She told me about her children. *All* of her children. Over a period of about seven or eight years, she had a series of pregnancies. Some ended in abortions, others in adoptions. One child was being raised by his biological father. Of course, her story, as she poured out her soul, was more than about her lost children—it was also about promiscuity, and abortion, and her profound sense of shame and guilt.

From the outset, she knew what she wanted to do to help to alleviate her spiritual anguish. She asked me to go with her to the local cemetery, where we would give each of her babies—and her past—a proper burial. We would together meet the pain, and through a holy ritual, let it go into God's loving hands.

A few days later, I met Melissa and a couple of her family members at Babyland, a small lot at the cemetery that holds the graves of perhaps thirty or more little ones. For the most part, they're here together because their parents didn't have family lots on which to bury their young 'uns, probably because they never envisioned having to bury their babies. I know a bit about this—Fran and I lost our third son at just seven weeks of age.

On that chilly October day, Melissa and I huddled together and read from Scriptures. She named her babies—"Sunday," "Monday," "Tuesday," "Wednesday," "Thursday," "Friday." We offered prayers for each one. We started with the *De Profundis* of Psalm 130: "Out of the depths I cry to you, O Lord. Lord hear my voice." And then we read Isaiah 43: "Do not fear, for I have redeemed you; I have called you by name, you are mine." We closed with a few psalms. Psalm 90, "Lord you have always been our home" and Psalm 139, "O Lord, you have searched me and known me. . . . Where can I go from your spirit?" It was a very sacred and profound moment for each one of us.

Jesus was in the graveyard that day. His feet were dirty from the dry sand kicking up on the road to Calvary. He stopped to meet his mother, to gaze into her eyes. Each of the babies—those nascent spirits that lived a brief time on this earth—looked up and met his or her mother for the first time. It was brief but grace filled. It was painful but redemptive. In that prayerful exchange in the graveyard, Jesus's eyes met the woman who gave birth to him. The encounter may have lasted no longer than a minute, and yet it accomplished a miracle.

In loving someone like Melissa, we may be tempted to feel like the parents of the *prodigal son*, worrying endlessly as we hope and pray that everything is all right. We can only imagine the pain of the parents of that young man who must have seemed, after all their love and nurture, to be lost for good.

We may be tempted to add up our *losses*, consider ourselves the victims of cruel fate, and take on the awesome burden of self-pity, which, in turn, is a plea to others for their pity. If we take this track, *losers* like us sound pretty pathetic, don't we?

For my entire adult life, I have turned again and again to a little bit of poetic wisdom from Alfred Lord Tennyson, who wrote in *In Memoriam*: "I hold it true, whate'er befall; I feel it, when I sorrow most; 'Tis better to have loved and lost, than never to have loved at all."

We've heard the last line so often that we mutter it in our sleep to anyone who runs into relationship problems. But for someone like myself, who has parented dozens of children, I can say with confidence that the risk of loving someone—and especially loving a person with a serious mental illness—has always been accompanied by gifts that are unexpected and unimaginable.

We could do some hard calculations, consider the

risk of reaching out to love another child, and decide not to do so when we count the cost of yet more parenting. But our faith argues persuasively against that exercise, because we know that our love is only a reflection of God's love and that God will never withhold from us the resources we need to be good parents.

We believe that God's love bridges life and death, and, in fact, gives life again after death. That's what happens on the road to Calvary, and I witnessed it happen in Babyland.

Simon of Cyrene Helps Jesus Carry the Cross

Scott Rose

Simon was a passerby who was pressed into service by the Romans to carry Jesus's cross. Like Simon, many families are drafted by biology to share their loved one's burden of mental illness, and they do so with heroic grace. But Walter is unlike anyone I've met. He was a passerby like Simon who *freely* chose to carry another's cross for a lifetime.

The first psychologist licensed in the state of Tennessee in the early 1950s, Walter worked in academia as a college professor and quickly earned a national reputation as an educational psychologist. With a little time on his hands as a thirty-year-old bachelor, Walter volunteered to do educational testing in a county-run orphanage. Every weekend, caring citizens of the area

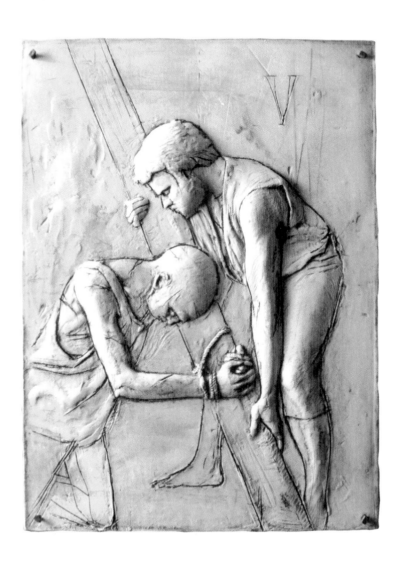

would come to visit some of the children and sometimes take them out for small trips. Many of the children had such sponsors—except ten-year-old Fred. I suspect it was because of the boy's mental health issues that no one chose to visit him. One day when Walter was volunteering there, Fred approached him and asked him to take him out for the day. Water could hear the cry below the request and responded. Immediately, Fred asked to stay overnight with Walter, and then later, begged to be adopted.

As a mental health professional, Walter fully understood the cross he was choosing to bear by raising the boy. But he did it anyway. And it was, indeed, a difficult journey. Loving a person with a mental illness takes a toll on the body, like caring for anyone with disabilities. However, compounded by the physical exhaustion is the mental anguish of worry, fear, guilt—and sometimes anger. In that regard, the family member or helper shares the same type of pain as the loved one.

Walter and Fred's journey was challenged from the start. Even though no other person was willing to adopt Fred, the local county social service office opposed the adoption because some artificial rules at the time determined it was inappropriate for a single man to adopt a boy. Walter had to engage an attorney to fight this first battle. Fortunately, the wise judge ruled in favor of the boy and his new father. But how discouraging that must have been to the man—to be willing to assume such a responsibility, and yet have to fight for it—when no one else wanted the child.

Walter and Fred created a good life together, and after ten years, Walter married a wonderful woman who had plenty of room in her heart to love Fred, too. But the challenge of loving a person with serious mental illness continued. Fred struggled through high school and college, handicapped by his shyness and emerging paranoia. Forever devoted to Fred, Walter tried to find the balance between always being there for Fred and yet at the same time encouraging independence. A former student of Walter's helped Fred get hired by an inner city African American high school in Washington, DC, to teach art to special education students, many with emotional disabilities. Having been raised in a small, all-white town in Tennessee, Fred landed in a foreign culture with significant challenges ahead of him. Petrified by the circumstances, Fred was too humble and accepting to complain or judge. Instead, he just worked hard. The principal once told Walter that while Fred was not the most skilled teacher at the school, he was the only one willing to do for the children whatever was asked of him.

Eventually full-blown schizophrenia emerged in Fred, and he became psychotically paranoid. As was always the case in Fred's life, Walter stepped in to help, and brought Fred back to live with him and his wife, and connected him to a wonderful psychotherapist who then moved to Frederick, MD. Fred expressed an interest in following him so that he could return to the Washington, DC, area. So the therapist connected Fred with Way Station, and we served Fred for twenty years. But even with all our support, Fred continued to rely on Walter as his lifeline, calling him several times each day—twenty times when he was anxious. Fred drove home to visit Walter every weekend. And Walter did the long drive whenever Fred requested his support, regardless of how small the need or how psychotic the paranoia. This was especially hard on Walter when he entered his eighties and was living with prostate cancer. His health and energy waned, but his fidelity to Fred continued unbending, like the beam of a cross.

Walter was always there for Fred. Always.

The average life span of a person with serious mental illness is twenty-five years shorter than that of the general population—due to a combination of psychiatric medications (with side effects that can cause diabetes and obesity), lack of skills and motivation to adopt healthy lifestyles, and a disproportionate prevalence of smoking. Fred was no exception. Last year, at age sixty-eight, Fred was fighting for his life in a Washington hospital for seven days with complications of a triple bypass surgery. Despite his own failing health at age eighty-five, Walter could not stay away. He drove or flew to Washington every couple of days. I would pick him up at the airport or drive him halfway home. Despite my protests, he insisted on sleeping each night on a cot in the janitor's closet next to the Intensive Care Unit, often being awakened early in the morning by housekeeping staff.

Fred passed away on July 4, 2014, and Walter has never fully recovered from the grief of this loss and a lifetime of pain.

I really believe Walter is a saint. Like so many other unsung heroes who love people with mental illness, he would resist that label. He would say that any person who had listened to that ten-year-old orphan would have done the same—pressed into service like Simon of Cyrene by a sense of duty. Interestingly, a Hebrew translation of the name Simon is "he who has heard." It would be wonderful if more people would have the kindness and humility to really listen to people with mental illness. Even in times of disorganized or psychotic thoughts, they have wisdom to share and love to give. But it is the saint like Walter who *hearkens,* hearing the cry and responding out of compassion.

Walter might concede that he was a good listener to Fred, but he would quickly add that he received as much from Fred as he gave to him, that there is nothing heroic in choosing to love someone, even if you know the road will be hard. There was a special strength and wisdom in that ten-year-old orphan that inspired him to reach out to Walter, a man who had everything—except someone who needed his love. I once asked Fred why he chose Walter. He smiled softly and said, "Dad and me, we had a connection."

Fred was a kind man who was generous with others and treated everyone with respect, regardless of status, race, intelligence, or disability. I can imagine how Fred's gentle humility and naiveté must have been a profound blessing to Walter who struggled against the arrogance and cynicism of academia. More importantly, though, Fred opened up Walter's heart at a critical time. A product of the Depression, Walter was a deprived and lonely child with two emotionally distant parents. His father was absent much of his childhood, and his mother worked twelve hours each day. Walter left home when he was seventeen to fend for himself, and he never returned. He remained a self-reliant bachelor until the age of thirty, when he adopted Fred, and forty when he married. He may never have been able to be vulnerable to another person had young Fred not modeled that for him, reaching out and asking for Walter's love.

Walter saved Fred. But Fred probably redeemed Walter.

Walter and I attended Fred's memorial service at Way Station together. We were both surprised to hear how many lives Fred touched with his unique blend of kindness, simplicity, and compassion. Through beautiful stories about Fred shared with me in the days afterward, and by grieving with Walter in months after, I grasped the depth and mutuality of their love. And I came to realize that finding each other was not a random passing.

I do believe Walter made a saintly choice in carrying Fred's cross. But I also think Fred carried Walter's. And is still doing so.

Veronica Wipes the Face of Jesus

Fred Wenner

In our church, a long-standing tradition has held that young children can't receive communion (the Eucharist) because they don't understand what it's all about. Our practice has been to have older children enroll in catechetical instruction where they learn all about the church and the sacraments. Once they are thus prepared and then confirmed, they will be qualified to come to the Lord's Table and enter into "the innermost sanctuary of the whole Christian worship."

However, more than twenty years ago, some church members began to challenge this historic practice and its rationale. Several had come into our congregation from churches that allowed children to receive communion, and when they learned that their children were

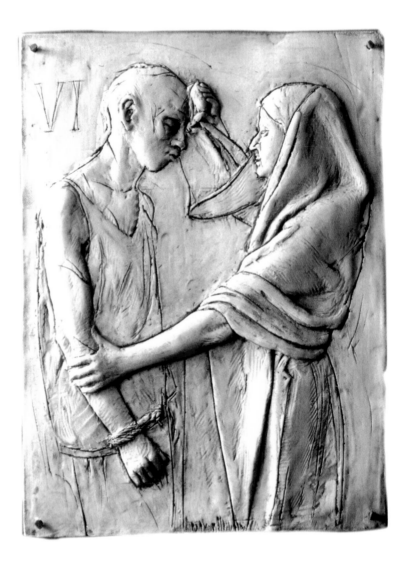

not welcome at our communion services, they were not silent about this perceived affront. So we developed a congregational study within which this hot-button issue was debated by members with differing perspectives. Eventually we were all reminded that Eucharistic liturgies call communion a *holy mystery*, which suggests that even intellectually brilliant adults are not expected to fully understand exactly how the sacraments convey the grace of God to the faithful.

Playing into that emerging consensus was the recollection of how moving it was for the congregation to witness the confirmation of our daughter Rachael, just a few years earlier. Those present knew of Rachael's struggles with serious mental illness that exacerbated the effects of her developmental disability. Did the church make a mistake in granting an exception and confirming Rachael when she certainly did not understand communion? Providentially, the church had made the right decision in confirming Rachael, and in 1994, we changed our policy to welcome all to the Lord's Table, whether or not the sacrament of God's grace was fully understood by the communicant.

While the confirmation/communion controversy was resolved without inflicting undue pain upon our daughter, there was another incident that proved to be even more painful, even excruciating.

When Rachael was old enough to qualify, she told us

that she wanted to give blood as I had done countless times. We targeted a particular place and time for our visit to the Red Cross bloodmobile, and we spent considerable time going over the particulars of the process of donating blood. Fran, my wife, and I talked with her about how much the gift of blood would mean to people with critical injuries and diseases. Rachael's steadfast desire to donate her blood evolved from her authentic humanitarian instincts. By the day of the bloodmobile visit she was ready and eager. We went together to give blood, father and daughter.

When we arrived at the bloodmobile site, I went first so she could see how it was done. Then I went back to Rachael and began to accompany her through the intake process. As they took her health history, I realized that our plan was already in jeopardy. Rachael simply did not understand most of the health questions they asked her.

When Rachael does not understand a question, she will usually reply with words like "I'm not sure." As she responded this way to question after question, she must have seemed to the nurse to be dismissive, because it was clear that the nurse was becoming increasingly frustrated by not being able to get the basic information.

I suggested that if the questions were framed more simply, Rachael would then be able to give appropriate answers. The nurse didn't know how to simplify. Instead she told us that Rachael could not give blood. I tried again to salvage the situation, this time asking to serve as a go-between, or interpreter, for Rachael. This too was rejected, and we had to leave.

I will never forget our drive home that day. Rachael did not verbalize her disappointment, at least not until we got into the car. Once the doors were shut in our safe cocoon, however, my daughter began to sob in a way that startled me, with an intensity that must have held years and years of her frustration. In that awkward moment, her profound suffering was breaking through to the surface, and I sat there helpless. It was deep, gut-wrenching, almost primal wailing that I had never heard before, nor have I heard since. Her pain made me sick to my stomach, even to my very soul, and this un-controlled explosion of her profound hurt has haunted me ever since. I saw in Rachael an awesome agony, not unlike the suffering of Christ, and I wanted somehow to mop up and dry her tears, just as Veronica did for Jesus shortly before his death.

For the next few days I made numerous phone calls, eventually talking to the doctors at the regional blood center who administer the program and set the rules. I tried to argue that anyone with a language problem would be offered an interpreter, and such an interpreter for Rachael should be allowed. The doctors were unre-lenting. She was denied the privilege of donating her blood because of her mental retardation.

Rachael joined our family when she was just four years old. She didn't like to wear clothes, she had no bathroom habits, and she didn't speak intelligibly. Early on, there was the question of whether the cause of her mental retardation was genetic or environmental. Several times since, evaluations have raised the possibility of autism. Whatever the cause of her difficulties, she was a gift to us—not from the foster care system, but from God. We regard *all* of our children as gifts from a gracious and loving God.

When she was young she seemed, at times, to struggle with how she fit in. One day, after an afternoon swim at a local pool where we had a family membership, she told us at dinner that she noticed that when each of the kids presented their cards at the gate, everyone had the name of Wenner . . . except for her. And then she just blurted out, "Why can't I be a Wenner too?" With no hesitation, we began the process of adoption, and Rachael became a happy camper.

Looking back on that event, I have only recently surmised that this may have been Rachael's way of asking for parity within the Wenner family—and perhaps even pleading, "Am I not a child of God . . . too?"

As Rachael reached her mid-twenties, the mental illnesses seen clearly in her biological parents began to manifest themselves in Rachael, as she developed schizoaffective disorder and obsessive compulsive disorder (OCD). The symptoms of both made her resistant to treatment and resentful of the help of some caregivers, including her parents, and the relentless mental illnesses with which she has been contending have taken their toll on her behavior and, to some extent on her sense of self-esteem. For Rachael, and so many others who often buckle under the weight of mental illness, there is consolation in the companionship of the one who had to trudge uphill to Calvary with a heavy burden, that ominous wooden cross, that he didn't deserve.

Despite her often cheery disposition and nonjudgmental demeanor, she was dogged by others' perceptions of her. The term *mental retardation* seemed to stick mercilessly. At the 1995 awards luncheon for the state-wide Maryland AAMR (explained to us as the American Association for people with Mental Retardation), Rachael was named the Outstanding Consumer. This gave her an opportunity to make an amazing personal and public statement.

With microphone in hand, she said to the large assembly: "When I learned that I had won this award, I was excited and proud. But as I read my letter, I could see and hear only one word, 'retarded.'" Rachael used her brief time at the podium to address the hurtfulness of that term, and she asked those present to think about what it would be like to "walk in my shoes." It was an event that unintentionally, but cruelly, highlighted her disabilities. Yet, with a courageous boldness, Rachael stood proud and spoke her truth. She showed that she was more than worthy of her award.

Today Rachael is not the person she once was. She's not always the gregarious, trusting, joyful child we raised years ago. Thankfully, she has had a Veronica here and there to lighten her load, to wipe away her tears, just like that day she wept in the car after being denied the chance to give blood. A dedicated cadre of caregivers has worked overtime to stabilize her tumultuous life. Her home includes 24/7 on-site supervision and a routine with which Rachael is thriving. She also has a meaningful work regimen at Way Station, where she interacts with other club members and receives constant support and affirmation from the staff. She sweeps every day everywhere, rakes leaves in the fall, and shovels snow in winter. She is fastidious beyond belief, and she loves her work more than anyone I know.

As parents, we've been through hell and back with Rachael, relentlessly advocating for appropriate school placements for her, fighting for safe working conditions for her, desperately seeking to understand and counteract the destructive impulses of her OCD, agonizing over numerous failed attempts to allow her to achieve greater independence, and going to court in a neighboring state in order to free her from an unscrupulous family that had exploited and degraded her.

What is the value of a person deemed less than worthy because of disabilities and limitations not of her choosing? This has seemed to be Rachael's lifelong question, and it's a question that lingers for me as well. One way to make sense of this seeming senselessness is to look back, or up, to the cross . . . to the moments when Jesus carries our burdens for us to his crucifixion, when all suffering is redeemed and love and hope are possible again even in the midst of illness. And if we're lucky, we meet a few Veronicas along the way.

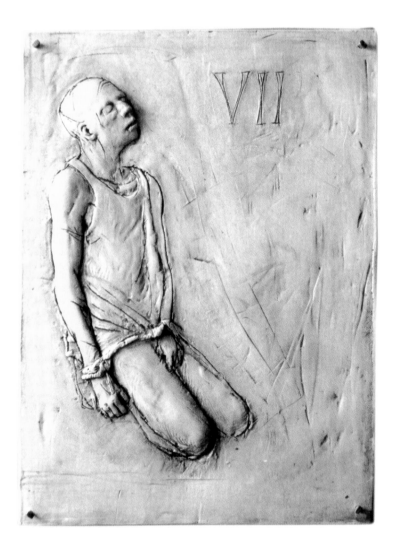

Jesus Falls the Second Time
Al Rose

Brenda was a graying, middle-aged woman carrying too much weight on her arthritic knees. She hobbled around with a cane. I first met her in the world culture's class, which many of the clients with a college background, like her, attended. Brenda was bright, with a wry sense of humor, especially in making comments about the US political scene when comparisons to other governments came up. She saw our virtues, and she saw our faults. And she expressed her opinions without hesitation, with a sort of glee.

Her illness manifested itself in bouts of schizophrenia. As odd as it seemed for a woman of her age, she carried around rag dolls in her big purse. They were dressed in polka-dot jumpers, with hair fashioned from thin strips of cloth. She would pull them out to introduce them to you, speaking for them, and nuzzling them. They were her children and her closest companions. Sadly, she was one of those many clients who had no relatives or close friends in the area. The ever-present static in the lives of most clients makes it too difficult for them to form close relationships. The unpredictability that is so often attached to severe mental illnesses constantly disturbs the soil needed for deep friendships to grow.

Somehow, she found out that I was Catholic and seemed to take pleasure in the knowledge that we were co-religionists. We would exchange casual comments about holy days and Catholic customs and practices. I enjoyed that. Many of the clients knew, somehow, that I was a clergyman, although I didn't wear the collar at Way Station. I suppose that some had seen me in the collar at a nearby coffee shop, taking a break during pastoral visits for my parish. But most were from Protestant sects. They were decent, often quite devout folk. Brenda, my co-religionist, was different.

A key moment in my experiences with Brenda occurred one year during Lent. She came to me, somewhat distressed, confiding that she wanted to go to reconciliation—although, at her age, she used the older term *confession*. The problem was that she was unable to get to the church near her during the regular hours for reconciliation. What to do? I advised her to call the church office and inquire if the priest could see her at another time. She had already done so, but the secretary had been hesitant, obviously trying to protect her over-worked pastor, one priest in a large parish, as is so often the case today. She had suggested that perhaps Brenda could call some other parishes to see if their times fit her schedule better. But for Brenda, public transportation posed serious difficulties, and no nearby parishes were directly on transit routes. And she didn't have the money for a sizable cab fare.

I then offered to check the parish close to our facility and, because I would not, as a volunteer, be allowed to transport her myself, I offered also to find a counselor who might run her over to the church during the work day. She was quite happy with that, and so I visited the parish. I felt that if their regular hours for reconciliation did not occur during the time Brenda was at the facility, I might be able to talk a priest into seeing her by appointment. It turned out that their hours did correspond to a time convenient for us. Then I found a counselor who would be willing to help. Pleased with myself for having found a solution to a problem, I presented the details to Brenda.

"Brenda!" I said, stopping her in the corridor. "Excellent news! The parish close to our facility is open for reconciliation, and I have found someone to help you get there!"

I expected her to jump up and down or hug me or

something. Instead her face froze. She seemed flustered. And she simply declined.

I was frustrated and irritated. Why had she decided not to go to reconciliation? Her answer was a confused mix of reasons stemming partly from her schizophrenia and partly because of the disapproving reaction of a person in her circle who was being very critical about it, and Brenda felt ashamed to go. How tempted I was to snap, "Why didn't you tell me about this sooner before I went to all this trouble?" Or, "What difference does it make what this person is saying? This is about your faith. It's your business, not hers!" Or even more severely, "Brenda, for heaven's sake, here it is Lent, and you said that you wanted to go to confession. So I went to all this trouble for you, and now you just brush it off! Are you really saying now that you do not need to go to confession?" But somehow (the Holy Spirit?), I just said, "Well, at least we now know how it can be worked out when you're ready."

I went away muttering to myself, quite exasperated. It was not unusual to meet with erratic responses from the clients. After all, our clients are dealing with severe mental illness, and as I said above, unpredictability is a predictable part of their conditions. That's part of the cross that they bear. Sometimes their therapy and their medicine work well, and they can begin relationships and fulfill responsibilities. But other times, those therapies do not work, and then these folks fall under that burden of the cross. It is sadly mysterious, like Jesus's Passion.

And that's what I needed to do: to place Brenda in the context of the Lenten story.

In the prisons, my spiritual role had been primarily that of presence. I might conduct services and talk with inmates interested in spiritual or religious questions, but mostly my job was what is called the ministry of presence. In a maximum-security prison, where most inmates have at least one life sentence, you are dealing with people who are so damaged by life that conversions are rare. Hopeless, bitter, angry, cynical, convinced of their own evil or worthlessness, many of these men needed one thing more than anything else: simple moments when they identified and experienced the goodness that still lay deep down in them. I sat with them in the yard and appealed, simply by my presence, to a sense that there was some worth in them. I knew that was what I could most do for them: to see Jesus in them and accompany him.

In prayer, I came to realize that my solving the problem of getting Brenda to reconciliation was not really that important. More critical was that she knew that she was precious in my eyes, that I was with her, that she was important enough for me to have extended myself in this way. My presence was the most valuable thing I could offer her, as it was to the inmates. She verified that many times thereafter by cheery, somewhat conspiratorial, greetings as we passed each other in the corridors, "Hello, friend." Yes, not a bad word for our relationship with Jesus!

But most importantly, I came to understand that I also needed to see Jesus in her, just as I had in the inmates in the prisons. I needed to accompany her on her difficult, painful journey, with its unavoidable falls. I realized it hadn't been her fault. My fault was in not seeing Jesus in her, falling under her burden.

I needed only to accompany Jesus along the Via Dolorosa and be with him there each time he falls.

Jesus Meets the Women of Jerusalem

Scott Rose

"A large crowd of people followed Jesus, including many women who mourned and lamented him. Jesus turned to them and said, 'Daughters of Jerusalem, do not weep for me; weep instead for yourselves and for your children'" (Luke 23:28).

I understood this story in a different way when I attended Allison's funeral. Suffering from schizophrenia and long-term institutionalization for decades, Allison was one of those tortured individuals for whom the illness, itself, prevented treatment. Paranoia and a secondary intellectual disability (formerly known as mental retardation) prohibited her from accessing traditional mental health counseling or from even taking her medication. Like a cancer feeding itself on good

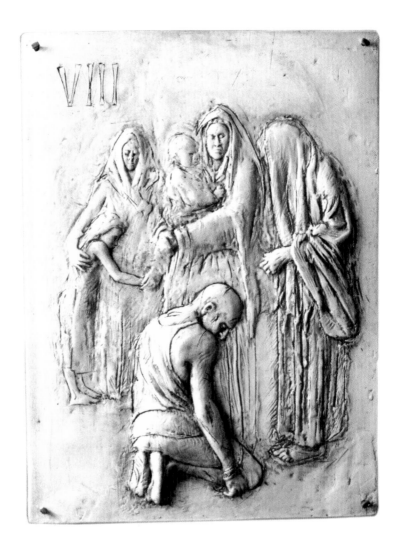

cells in order to grow, her mental illness prevented all possible forms of healing. She spiraled into the revolving door between hospitalization and homelessness, and then fell prey to exploitation and prostitution, grasping for love.

She also had medical problems, including incontinence, which started in her early forties, probably a traumatic response to childhood sexual abuse, and it grew progressively worse. But she didn't seem to care and didn't have the desire or the means to prevent it by taking the medication prescribed by the urologist or even changing into clean clothes. Perhaps this condition subconsciously helped her, repulsing some perpetrators. Regardless, she was fine with sitting on plastic garbage bags in cars or chairs. She had little affect, numb to her tragic circumstances, and never seemed to get angry with people or life, although she often argued out loud with voices in her head. The memory I have of Allison is one of profound contrast—her sitting on a garbage bag in urine-soaked pants, with a broad, lovely smile that surely hid enormous pain but revealed a couple missing front teeth and a lot of endearing vulnerability.

At Way Station we refuse to yield to the insidious nature of mental illness. If the illness prevents the individual from coming to us, we go to the individual—on the streets, under the highway passes, and over to the tent communities in the woods. We doggedly tracked

down Allison through the modern-day brothels in all
their subtle forms, and we would reengage her in Way
Station's community.

For one or two days. Then back at it again. For a
decade.

When I heard Allison had died in the county nursing home, I wanted to go to the funeral to represent
her other community. I sat in the back of the African
American church, with a handful of women up front,
weeping quietly, and a few men and children in the
middle. I had the sense that no one really knew her
but that the mourning women were volunteer *wail-
ers* of the congregation, offering tears out of respect
for what few extended family were there. And no one
knew me or that Way Station had kept Allison alive
for ten years.

Then came one of the most unusual and loving eu-
logies I have ever heard. An elderly, physically disabled
woman struggled up to the altar and introduced herself as Allison's *aunt*—though it was clear that this was
not a blood connection. She went on to share her own
pain and her decision years ago to throw her husband
out because he would not choose her over alcohol. She
recalled one day when she went to check up on him in
his apartment during the separation and found Allison
sitting on his bed smoking a cigarette. Allison emphati-
cally denied the obvious—that she had been sexually

involved with the husband. The old woman quoted herself as replying, "It's OK, Allison. My husband and I will get things right someday. But for now, I'm just glad you are safe and off the streets."

My first reaction was to be filled with awe at the old woman's fidelity. One of the most overwhelming challenges in supporting people with mental illness is to sustain commitment to them, especially when the illness often creates resistance to that support—and in this case, outright betrayal. The woman shared that she continued to look out for Allison her entire life, even following her to an adjoining room in the same nursing home, continuing to provide chocolates—and friendship—until Allison died.

My second reaction came years later when I reflected on the scene in light of the Stations of the Cross. When I remember the old woman telling Allison not to worry about her but instead to take care of herself, I am reminded of Jesus telling the lamenting women not to weep for him but instead to weep for themselves. Both were selfless redirections of the greater cause for concern and the greater need for action.

Twenty years ago when I witnessed these words of compassion, I was moved by the purity and fidelity of the old woman's love. But now, looking back, I appreciate even more her wisdom in understanding what should be said and done. She realized that Allison deserved her support—which she had the ability to provide by opening up her heart—more than she deserved Allison's loyalty, which was prevented by a disease beyond Allison's control or culpability.

In a way, this *wailing* woman of Frederick was countering Jesus's rebuke. She could weep for herself *and* for the suffering Christ. No one would have blamed the old woman if she had terminated the friendship, but many of us marvel at her insight and compassion in choosing to continue to support Allison. I think we should cry for both of them.

And like Jesus's words, the old woman's go deeper, too. I would like to believe that she was also talking to the other mourning women at the funeral—and the larger community. By redirecting the women to weep for themselves, Jesus was expressing compassion for the community's general sinfulness and specifically for rejecting him. While I sometimes get angry with society's rejection of people with mental illness, this story reminds me that I should also feel compassion for society and its misguided fears. After all, few people are blessed with the wisdom and fidelity of that old woman. And, in the end, her life would have not been as rich or redemptive had she rejected Allison that day in her husband's apartment. She wouldn't have had anybody to give chocolates to. She was a nursing home resident who nurtured patients. I could tell when she spoke at the funeral that she felt centered and strong—and maybe even a little proud—with her response to Allison and her enduring commitment.

Jesus concludes his response to the women of Jerusalem by noting why he has more pity for them and their children then he does for himself:

> For indeed, the days are coming when people will say, "Blessed are the barren, the wombs that never bore and the breasts that never nursed." At that time people will say to the mountains, "Fall upon us!" and to the hills, "Cover us!" for if these things are done when the wood is green what will happen when it is dry? (Luke 23:29-31)

Jesus is prophesizing about the apocalyptic consequences of human sin at the end of time. But this passage and this station cause me to wonder sometimes whether a person like Allison who suffered such a tragic life—due in large part to society's neglect and sin—would have been better off if her mother had never bore her. Indeed, lessening some of her biological challenges might have only exacerbated the tragedy and evil around her. Had she been less cognitively impaired, she might have been more aware of and saddened by the injustice of her life. Had she been less incontinent, she might have been raped more often. It is easier to crucify with dry wood.

But then I remember the old woman's eulogy, and I realize that Allison's life inspired graced moments of redemption for others, including that old lady, the wailing women of Frederick—and me. And I recall the memory of Allison smiling on a garbage bag. I weep for everyone—out of sadness *and* joy.

NINTH STATION

Jesus Falls the Third Time
Scott Rose

Like many low-income people with severe mental illness, John fell multiple times in his life under the triple burden of disease, poverty, and discrimination. One of these elements alone has the power to extinguish the flame of hope inside a person with mental illness. As we have seen throughout the reflections in this book, so many people with severe mental illness are buried before their time, with a sparse crowd to grieve for them at their funeral. But unlike many tragic stories, John got back up and overcame fall after fall.

A significant part of the good fight on the journey of mental illness is dealing with the social dynamic of *not in my backyard*. And as with most battles, this struggle is complex. Generally, the potential neighbors are not mean people who are intentionally discriminating.

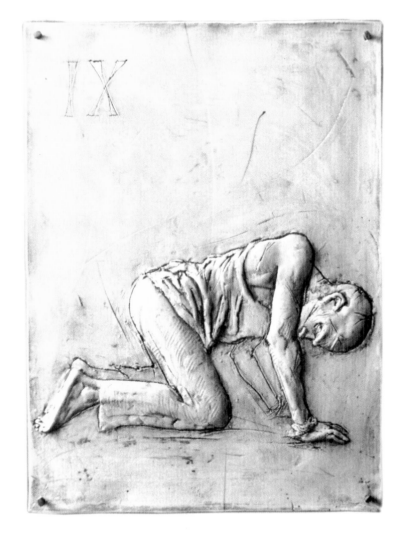

They are just afraid because of misperceptions tucked away somewhere in their minds.

In the early days of Way Station, though, one particular neighborhood united in angry and unkind ways to try to prevent us from moving in. While federal fair housing laws mandate neighborhoods to *tolerate* people with mental illness, the journey of recovery needs communities to *welcome* them.

It was in this context that John courageously chose to walk with his cross through a crowd who despised him and wanted to see him fall.

Within two days of our signing the real estate contract to purchase a house, several neighbors started handing out leaflets stating that Way Station clients would be moving in and would rob the neighborhood houses and sexually abuse the children. Local elected officials were contacted and asked to apply pressure, and several petitions were initiated. We were invited—rather, challenged—to come to a neighborhood meeting to hear the protest. Instead, we invited the neighborhood to come to us in our outpatient building to hear about who we were before they would have the opportunity to tell us who we were not.

For a solid week, all the staff and clients prepared for this reception. Clients baked cake and cookies, staff prepared presentations, friendly families and supportive citizens from other neighborhoods were invited as support. John, a long-time client with schizophrenia, offered to tell his story so that the neighbors could put a face to mental illness and learn who we really were. As with many people served by Way Station, John had a history of difficulties starting in adolescence: he fought depression, paranoia, addiction, social phobia, homelessness, and an occasional religious delusion in which he believed he was an angel and would wear all-white clothes instead of his usual blue jeans. His illness began to emerge at age seventeen when he was in Catholic school and started obsessing about faith. Then, full-blown psychosis set in, with unrelenting thoughts that the "eyes of the world" were glaring at him in judgment.

When the day came, everyone at Way Station was nervous, especially when steady streams of scowling neighbors flowed in, along with an elected official and a lawyer the neighborhood had hired. I began to second-guess our decision to allow John to speak, fearing for his emotional safety. He was a fragile man suffering from social phobia and paranoid delusions that people hated him, and he was about to put himself on the line in front of one hundred angry people who really did dislike him. I could see how nervous he was, and I reminded him that he didn't need to do it. But he insisted on going through with it, saying that it was important that the audience hear directly from someone with mental illness.

Discrimination can be one of the most overwhelming and discouraging of the three burdens—for the individual who is suffering *and* for the caregivers. With other illnesses, a person often gets sympathy and support. But discrimination breeds blame not compassion. Common symptoms of the disease include self-isolation, paranoia, and self-loathing, and public rejection exacerbates those symptoms. For all those suffering directly or indirectly, including family and caregivers, it is hard enough to battle the pain of illness and the limitation of poverty. But to also have to fight the shame of stigma can break you some days, slamming your head and your heart into the dirt. That day, as I looked at the angry crowd and knew it was time to start, I felt my knees buckle.

Several staff opened the presentation, discussing facts and misperceptions about mental illness and describing our program. I spoke a little bit about the federal fair housing laws, not as a sword, but rather as a shield to explain to the audience how it would be illegal for us to steer people with mental illness away from their neighborhood in the same way it would be illegal for us to do so with other minority groups. But it became clear pretty soon that the neighborhood wanted to fight, not listen. The frowns only grew more noticeable, and people started to fidget and sigh in frustration.

Then it was John's turn. He spoke eloquently of his

journey with mental illness, beginning with his troubled childhood, the emerging terror of the paranoid delusions, and the painful young adult years filled with homelessness and hospitalizations. And then, making himself vulnerable to a hate-filled crowd of one hundred people, he expressed his hurt in a soft, trembling voice: "If I was part of any other minority, you wouldn't assume that I would abuse your children . . . Why do you think I would do such a terrible thing just because I have mental illness?" He sat down, and the silence was deafening. Then, some clapping started, and before we knew it, a couple people were on their feet, applauding. Some neighbors who had come in angry were wiping tears from their eyes and apologizing for not understanding who we were. Several months later, Way Station moved into the house to a welcoming community.

When I reflect on this day, I marvel at John's courage and humility in publicly sharing the private pain of his life. He allowed himself to fall in front of a hateful crowd, like Jesus stumbling toward Calvary. I am inspired by his strength: after presenting his story, *he got back up* and confronted the crowd with the uncomfortable truth of their prejudice. And I recognize how his heroic act offered redemption for the neighbors who, in their defense, had left their hearts open enough to change and love rather than hang on to fear and anger.

On that day, in that moment, John was the holy figure he yearned in delusion to be.

Twenty years later, this neighborhood is one of our staunchest supporters, and because of them we experience less resistance as we move into other communities. After we spend time educating new neighborhoods and allaying some fears, they often ask for *references*—neighbors of other Way Station houses. We always direct them to the neighborhood that John walked through with his cross that day—in his blue jeans.

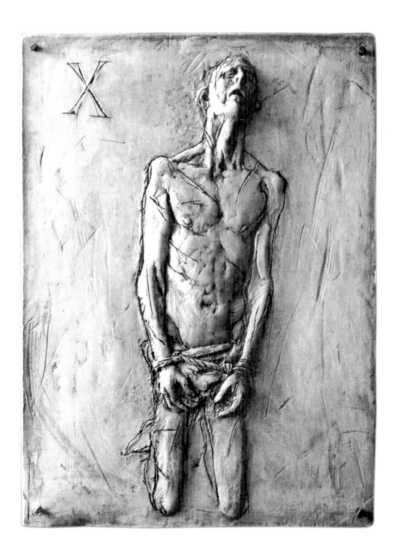

Jesus Is Stripped of His Garments

Al Rose

Patrick was one of the strongest human beings I have ever met. He had been stripped of a capability, suffered a profound loss, one that would have sunk many of us into self-pity. Not he.

From my own childhood through my early maturity, I had been vaguely uncomfortable with the only picture of Jesus that seemed prevalent, the Sunday-school portrait of him as a sweet, gentle teacher of good behavior. A Catholic should have known that there was more: the crucifix with the suffering Jesus hanging from it over the altar of every Catholic Church, the stations ranged down the two side walls, and the annual Lenten practice of walking with him every Friday night. But somehow that earlier picture from childhood had dominated my own view and discomfited me for many years. Perhaps for many like me, the extraordinary success of Mel Gibson's fierce, often brutal movie *The Passion of the Christ* was a powerful reminder of the Scripture's description of the Passion. I had personally discovered the Jesus of the Passion in my later maturity. But like Gibson's movie, Patrick was a startling reminder.

One rainy morning as I entered Way Station, there at the entrance, parked under the canopy in his wheelchair, was Patrick, both legs amputated at the knees. He had been an addict and on the streets. One time, in a stupor, he had fallen asleep in an alley, and flies had laid eggs in wounds on his legs. From that came maggots, from that a critical infection that required the amputations.

As I walked past him he said, "Good morning, Al, how are you?"

I had rushed to get there and was tired from other activities the day before, so I replied bravely, "I'm O.K., Pat, how are you?"

He replied, "Great."

The difference between his reply and mine stunned me. Mine laid bare to me my own lack of gratitude for what I have.

I never had occasion to converse with him again. We merely greeted each other in passing in the halls. But I have never forgotten that encounter. Today, as every day since, when someone asks me how I am, my reply is always, "Great," as it was in my hall encounters with him. I've thought often about that morning. It began a process of learning, first from Pat, then from another client at Way Station, Shirley. What I came to understand in a way that penetrated deeply was a special concept of poverty, which would lead me to a new insight about our Lord's Passion.

Sadly, Shirley suffered from paranoia. Tattooed, with long, stringy purple-streaked hair and wearing black leather clothes, she looked tough, probably an intentional, defensive pose, but, in fact, she was quite vulnerable. She believed that there were police plots against her, government plots, and even ones conjured by her relatives. Not an easy person in whom to find Christ.

She often stopped in a classroom where I was waiting for the period to start. She clearly wanted someone to listen to her. She talked of court cases and asked for advice. Of course, I could never give her any, just suggesting, I hope compassionately, that she needed a lawyer. Sometimes, she would just want to chat, ramble really. I think her paranoia isolated her, and she sought some contact, any contact, so long as it was kind.

One day, she had come into the office area where I had a desk and had perched on the edge of my desk, her face strained, to recount recent acts against her. She spent a good twenty minutes, telling me about those acts, by individuals, by businesses, by the government. I tried to listen patiently and sympathetically, until she finally concluded by proclaiming that she had proof. She then pulled out a stack of random cards, coupons, and passes, spread them out, and said, "See?" She looked at me intently and added, "You believe me, don't you?"

I don't know what a therapist would have said to her, but I'm not one. I just said, "Yes." The result in her was like the sun appearing suddenly from behind a cloud, a beautiful, beautiful smile. And then she left.

At the time, her smile did not register on me, because I was saddened by the extent of her paranoia, by those random cards and papers on the desk, and by the incoherence of her talk. But that night I couldn't get her smile out of my mind. In the moment of the smile, I had experienced consolation, the Ignatian sign of the presence of a loving God. And so I let it become the matter of my prayer.

I believed I had done the right thing in the way I had responded to her, but I was, nevertheless, a bit uncomfortable with the encounter. I knew it was because she represented a number of these folks with whom I had difficulty carrying on anything like a coherent conversation. As I offered it in prayer, I began to think of my time as a hospice chaplain. I had sat with dying people when words were just not important. And yet it had always been beautiful: I had experienced intense consolation. Why, I asked myself? I realized then that I had not listened to the hospice patients with my mind, but rather with my heart. I saw now that the folks like Shirley, struggling to communicate from their poverty of relationships, were not so different: their words were not so important, and I didn't need to be frustrated by them. I just needed to listen primarily with my heart.

Caryl Houslander, a spiritual writer of the last century, has a beautiful book on the Blessed Mother, *The Reed of God*. It is not just about Mary, though she is the focus; it is also filled with insights and poetic ways of expression about her son. One beautiful thought of hers struck me: she reminded me that we should recognize him not just as in Matthew 25, where we learn that the risen Christ can be found in the least of his people, in the poor, the stranger, the sick, the imprisoned. But Houselander pressed home for me the point that we can see Jesus, as well, in particular aspects of his life among us. Specifically here, I realized I was seeing Jesus during his Passion.

And I realized that I had met in Patrick and Shirley, two people who, even in their mental illness, mirrored Jesus as he was stripped on his way to the cross.

That realization became, in psalmist's words, "a light to my path." I saw that folks at Way Station have been stripped of almost everything that I had thoughtlessly accepted as I enjoyed the comforts of home and family, relationships, respect of friends, a future to which I could look forward.

What a gift from God is the beauty of poverty in those with mental illness, those who—like Jesus—have so little and yet can teach us so much.

How necessary it is for us to accompany Jesus in his Passion, stopping to recognize him whenever in our journey we see him stripped.

Jesus Is Nailed to the Cross
Scott Rose

Will's hands were nailed to his cross—by a pen. His schizophrenia began to emerge when he was a boy. The symptoms started with an obsessive delusion that he was getting smaller. Most troubling of all, he intentionally hurt himself by frequently puncturing his flesh with pens. After a long and painful struggle, he ended up living almost two years of his adolescence in a psychiatric hospital five hundred miles away from home.

However, the boy also heard a positive voice amidst the darkness of this illness: that of a muse. At the same time his illness began, he also felt deep within himself an inspiration to write poetry. Fortunately, he was willing to listen to that voice. It helped him find some

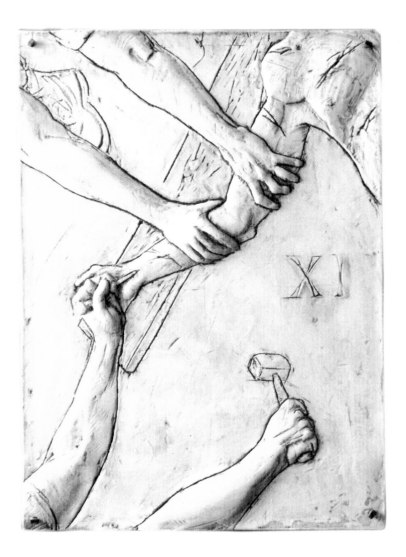

purpose and connection with the self he couldn't connect with otherwise, amidst the confusing thoughts and feelings. It helped him to survive the trauma of the lonely long-term hospitalization at a time in one's development when friends and family are critical. During transitional times when he was expelled from high schools, writing became his consistent friend and confidant. After graduating from college with honors and then some graduate degree coursework, he pursued the art more seriously and experienced success in publishing various poems and short stories. It helped him feel good about himself for the first time in his life.

This gift also helped him find his way in managing the symptoms of his mental illness. He tried going to Way Station, and that is where I met Will. For a while, Way Station was a good experience for him, but the paranoia and social anxiety associated with his particular illness ultimately made these group-based rehabilitation services unbearable for him, and after several years he stopped participating. But he maintained relationships with staff at Way Station by sending poetry and writing e-mails and cards. From the lonely place in his parents' basement, he found a way to stay connected with the world in intimate ways.

At the time Will first came to Way Station, I had come to another crisis point in my professional journey. I, and a couple other senior managers, had begun to feel tired and discouraged again, and we were just slogging through our days, seeing no hope and feeling no inspiration. A strange and blessed thing happened as a result of those cards, e-mails, and poems that Will sent us. I cannot explain exactly how it came about, but perhaps it was that his art, created from the same place as his mental illness, revealed the beauty in the disease and inspired hope in the struggle. In fact, Will was solely responsible for my starting to write again, as he and I collaborated on a fund-raiser essay contest. At any rate, it seems as if what he sent was graced through the Holy Spirit because my personal and professional depression, and that of some of my colleagues, lifted and we were able to reengage with new spark.

Psychosis is one of the symptoms of mental illness that can make it especially hard for caregivers to cope. The strangeness of it can be frightening to us, even when we do not feel physically threatened. And we can feel helpless and embarrassed trying to respond to it, and hopeless that our advice will not be heard or understood. In my relationship with Will, I found God even in psychosis.

This is not to say that Will is just wildly creative and does not also suffer from a psychotic disorder. He is both. Will needs his biweekly Prolixin shot so that he doesn't return to darker spaces. In fact, sometimes he wants to stop taking the medicine because he misperceives that it curbs his creativity. And while there can be a correlation between creativity and mental illness (e.g., Vincent Van Gogh, Ernest Hemingway, and most recently, Robin Williams), this correlation should not be glorified. Creativity is a gift, and mental illness is a painful disease.

However, it is to say that individuals with mental illness are much more than the illness—and sometimes they are gifted because of the illness. They can be ill and wise at the same time—psychotic and prophetic. And caregivers like me experience hope when we see dream in delusion, art in anguish, and call in hallucination.

Two years ago, Will's life was again traumatized when he found his father dead in the house after a fall. I went to the funeral, which was lovely, but I kept thinking that Will's poetry would have been more profound and healing than the Scriptures that were recited.

His elderly mother moved to Florida, but Will pleaded with his siblings to allow him to remain in Frederick. They reluctantly agreed to subsidize an apartment for him, with the condition that he receives case management services from Way Station. He recognized that he needed support without his parents, but he was ambivalent about reconnecting formally. In the end he agreed, and a staff person visits him in his apartment each week to check in. I, on the other hand, am honored to be in more frequent contact with him, corresponding with him through e-mail, as he sends me copies of his recent writings or expresses his thoughts and reflections—some paranoid, some anxious, but all articulate and wise. We have maintained a friendship through e-mail for over a decade, and I hope that we can continue that for the rest of our lives.

The greatest gift of my friendship with Will was made known to me in a recent insight I had while reflecting on his life in the context of this station. I realized that the very thing that represents Will's psychosis also symbolizes his spiritual calling. He used a pen to puncture his flesh when his illness surfaced as a child, and he used a pen to pursue his spiritual calling to poetry as an adult—a calling that has shone beauty amidst the darkness to me and many other people.

And he uses this same pen to help him manage his mental illness. In his poem below, Will personifies his illness as a demon that he fights through the night but that, in the surrender of morning, he recognizes to be an angel. Through this piece, Will articulates the terror of mental illness and finds hope.

Jacob and the Angel
By Will Mayo

At night I wrestle with the demon,
a long horned invisible monster

with steel-tipped claws
and fangs made out of ivory.
His wings are of feather and lace,
and reach from star to star
across the cloudy night.
And he is known only
by the breadth of his touch,
between which
he feels the cracks of the soul.
I snore all too loudly for this beast,
and turn from sheet to sheet
across the confines of my bed.

In the morning,
my nails will be red
with the touch of my blood.
And the beast with whom I have wrestled
will be known
only by the scratch upon my thigh,
the cry of a lost soul within,
and the crawl of a ladder to heaven.
The sores of an angel
are far too near for human flesh.

Like the Cross, a pen for Will represents both suffering and redemption.

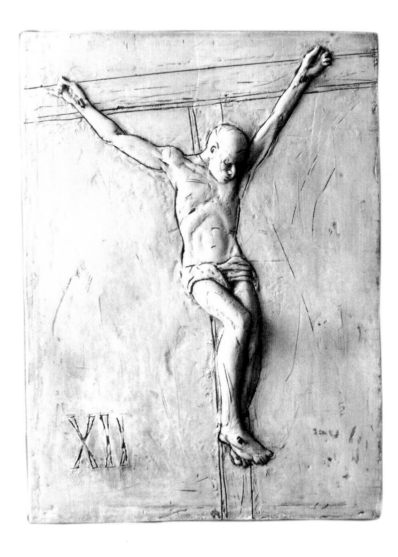

Twelfth Station

Jesus Dies on the Cross
Fred Wenner

In October of 1996, I attended a vigil in downtown Frederick, an annual gathering that marks Mental Illness Awareness Week. There I had an epiphany about depression and suicide. As I listened to the speakers on the steps of the county courthouse, candle in hand, I thought about our foster son Kevin. He had spent two years with us in our home in Pennsylvania until he graduated from high school, joined the Marines, and soon left for Vietnam.

When Kevin came home from the war, he went to the Marine base at Cherry Point, North Carolina. A few months later, he put his M16 to his head and pulled the trigger. The Marines chalked it up to accidental death while he was cleaning his rifle, but his best friend from high school days was with him in the barracks that night, and he told us that Kevin had been depressed and that his death was a deliberate, self-inflicted act.

Fran, my wife, and I had never really dealt with Kevin in terms of his depressive or manic behavior. We remember how, at times, he had far too much unbridled, mischievous energy than our well-ordered household could tolerate. At other times, Kevin became somber and emotionally withdrawn. In the 1960s, when we were in our twenties, we weren't schooled to look for some of the well-defined signs of mental illness that we are now taught to discern. We were not relating to him clinically. Nor at the time did we have a Way Station. For better or for worse, we were his parents, and our only instinct was to embrace him as a member of our family.

In a way, it's not surprising that at that mental illness vigil twenty-four years after his death, I realized for the first time that Kevin had had a hefty case of depression and that he had probably been bipolar. More startling for me personally was my sudden awareness that I was the father of a suicide victim, a realization that gave me permission to grieve in a different way than I did at his untimely death in 1972. Almost a quarter of a century later, there I stood at the foot of Jesus's cross, asking for the strength to grieve the life of my son, whose agony was more than he could bear.

After Kevin's tour of duty in Vietnam, in the months between his return to the states and his tragic death, he was visiting us at home and he asked me pointedly, "Why do you do what you do . . . taking in children and that?"

My reply was a halting, "Well, we just . . . like . . . figure it's what we're supposed to do." Fortunately, he didn't press me for a better explanation, because I know I fumbled my answer. I didn't want to seem too pat and pious, so I just talked in generalities, not specifically about my *calling* but about the need of all of us to help and care for one another. Toward the end of our little sit-down, I very pointedly said, "You know, we love you, Kevin . . . very much." I guess that if that's all he might have remembered, that's good, and our chat was useful.

Still, I've always had some difficulty answering Kevin's question, posed over the years by many people in many different ways. The question goes beyond the choice to accept a foster child with special needs. It also applies to the decision parents of biological children with mental illness must make each day regarding why and how to keep loving and working in spite of the challenges and despair. As Fran and I have struggled to find a good way to speak about our motivations, we have always seemed to begin by noting that we were both raised in families where love was abundant and our parents joyously modeled Christian generosity and hospitality.

Because of this grace-filled upbringing, our motivating spirituality is really second nature to us—more properly, it's probably our first nature. We just assume the working of God in our lives and relationships, and we don't expend much effort trying to define it or convey it in words. The love of God and the love of family are simply, yet profoundly, the very cradles in which we were rocked as infants and the very essence of our senses and sensibilities as our family is shaped and reshaped over our lifetimes. Beyond that, we simply trust that our spiritual underpinnings, so natural to us, are naturally self-evident to others.

So we naturally offered that love, and in 1967, Kevin was one of our first foster children to join our family. The circumstances were not terribly unusual. He had run afoul of the law, was tagged as a *juvenile delinquent*, and was about to be sent to a state *reform school.*

At that point, the authorities offered him an alternative. Instead of going away to a juvenile prison, he was told that he could join a foster family and receive something akin to supervised probation. Kevin opted for the latter, considering it the least of two evils. From the day he arrived at our home, Kevin called me *warden* and always referred to Fran as *warden's wife*—seemingly harsh names, but understandable preferences for this sixteen-year-old, given his very limited options.

In many ways Kevin was a delight, although he needed constant watching and strict supervision. Once, he arrived home to announce that he had just bought a car from a friend for something like $50. He was well shy of eighteen and didn't even have a driver's license, but neither of those facts had seemed to register with him. He had been on some kind of a high and was soaring above such banalities, so we had to bring him back down to earth.

On another occasion, again when his mind seemed a bit detached from reality, he took all the mice he was raising in his room, put them in a round cookie tin, and then rolled the tin down a sloping concrete walkway in the backyard. Obviously, we had to have a talk with Kevin about how we need to care more humanely for all of God's creatures.

At other times Kevin seemed despondent and was withdrawn, often retreating to the safety of his room, which held his few, but familiar, possessions. Knowing that teenagers need a certain degree of privacy, we respected his need to close his door and shut us out. It was never done with demonstrable malice, and we took no offense. But we worried a bit about his down times.

And then there were the more mellow times when he was comfortable enough to be completely enmeshed in our normal family activities. He loved to interact with our two young sons, then only two and three years old. They'd climb into his lap and swarm all over him, and his caring for them was often seen in his sly smile and his gentle patience with the little pests. He'd sing softly to them when they were settling down for the night—his favorite song was Simon and Garfunkel's "At the Zoo." And sometimes his feelings were expressed in cryptic notes, written in chalk on a small stool, chiding the youngsters for their bad aim when they stood to pee in the bathroom they all shared.

When our third biological son was born in the summer of 1968, Kevin was fully a member of the Wenner family and he definitely enjoyed the little "furd," as he called him—I never figured out exactly how he came up with that word. Tragically, just seven weeks after our handsome and healthy young son was born, he died suddenly one Saturday night. The doctors at the hospital worked feverishly for several hours to slow down the beating of his heart as it raced inexplicably and eventually wore him out. They pronounced our dead son a victim of SIDS—Sudden Infant Death Syndrome—which was really a way of saying that they had no idea why this happened to him.

In the hectic days following our baby's death, Kevin clearly was grieving, although we seemed to grieve apart. While we were attending to all of the arrangements and dealing with the anguish of other family members, Kevin was often quietly and lovingly watching over our other two sons. We may not have ever told him how much we appreciated all that he did during those tumultuous times. Nor did we ever ask him the question that he posed to us: with all the pain he had to deal with in his life, why—how—did he do what he did for our family?

I wish I could have also understood, on a somewhat spiritual level, why Kevin did what he did for his country. Not surprisingly, Kevin and I had some serious disagreements, perhaps more than would normally and naturally exist between a father and a son. The biggie was over the Vietnam War. I was standing on street corners getting signatures on petitions to end the war, and on occasion I would be on the mall in Washington, DC, at the larger demonstrations. Kevin looked forward to becoming a Marine because it held out for him the best hope of doing something truly significant, and, who knows, maybe even sacrificial. We would argue about the war strenuously, but not heatedly, and our differences did not destroy our relationship. In fact, those arguments may have strengthened our bond because we learned to respect each other's needs and perspectives.

Now, of course, I could harbor many regrets. And to be honest about it, I probably still do. What if I had put my foot down and forbade him from joining the armed forces? What if he had never been to Vietnam—would his depression have been less than lethal, absent his harrowing and haunting experiences there? What if we knew he had posttraumatic stress disorder? What if we could have gotten him to a Way Station? What if? What if? Did all the people surrounding Jesus the day of his crucifixion ask the same questions? Did they think that if they loved him in a different way, they could have spared him the humiliation and agony of the cross? Two young men in the prime of their lives—could, or should, anything have been done to keep them from meeting their untimely and undeserved deaths? What if? What if?

Over the years we learned to love Kevin very deeply. Actually, it wasn't very surprising at all that we would take to the good-looking blonde-haired guy, given the way he participated in our family life. And it wasn't long before we began to regard our strange names, *warden* and *warden's wife*, as terms of endearment. We still do, and the occasional recollection of the sound of those words from Kevin's lips continues to be a source of consolation in the decades since his death.

It took twenty-four years after Kevin's death for me to identify myself as a father of a suicide victim. It took fourteen years after that realization before I was able to begin to articulate, in spiritual terms, the reason I had chosen to love the child I then lost.

The twelfth station would be the one featured in a trailer if Jesus's life were an Academy Award–winning film. It's the pinnacle, the holiest of moments, if you consider his death the beginning of the paschal mystery that frees us to love more fully as human beings, that allows us to open our hearts to welcome a child into our home, a child who has the freedom to take his own life.

For Fran and me, the love embodied in Jesus's sacrificial death offers us the strength and the courage to pursue the directions of the resurrected Jesus.

In the last chapter of the Gospel of John, Jesus shares fish and bread with his disciples, cooked over a charcoal fire on the beach. As foster parents, we have always loved this dialogue:

> When they had finished breakfast, Jesus said to Simon Peter, "Simon son of John, do you love me more than these?" He said to him, "Yes, Lord; you know that I love you." Jesus said to him, "*Feed my lambs.*" A second time he said to him, "Simon son of John, do you love me?' He said to him, "Yes, Lord; you know that I love you." Jesus said to him, "*Tend my sheep.*" He said to him the third time, "Simon son of John, do you love me?" And he said to him, "Lord, you know everything; you know that I love you." Jesus said to him, "*Feed my sheep.*" (John 21:15)

Purely and simply, if we love Jesus, we will care for his lambs. And because of the twelfth station, we have the strength and the mandate to do so. That's our final answer to Kevin's searching question. We know that he's hearing us now.

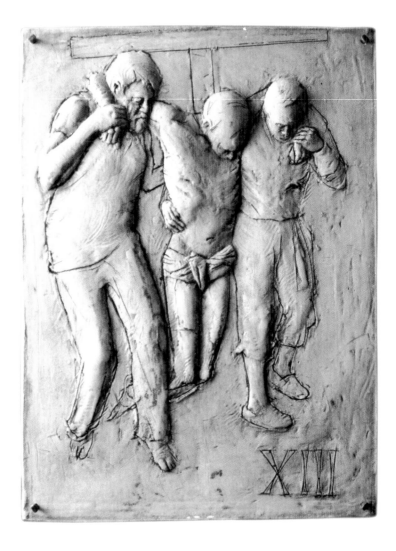

Jesus Is Taken Down from the Cross

Scott Rose

Dave was a Vietnam veteran with raging mental illness, raging alcoholism, and a raging mother. Dave seemed destined to remain in the back wards of the local Veterans Administration hospital. At twenty-three years old, I was Dave's counselor, and I resented him and his mother. He fought Way Station every step of the way to avoid treatment, and his mother badgered us to force treatment. Things culminated with Dave assaulting another employee, and I testified against him in court. And yet, despite all of this, the saintly director of Way Station urged me to keep trying with Dave.

I was too young to appreciate fidelity, much less that level. Dave's assault, compounded by his mother's insults, threw me over the edge. So I tried to sabotage

Dave's participation with Way Station by calling his mother's angry bluff each time she threatened to fire us. I gave up on Dave, wanting him to be taken down from his cross and hidden out of my sight—in the tombs of some institution.

I was making the same mistake as some communities do. We want to hide those who are most disabled—move them out of the city, away from businesses and neighborhoods, so that we don't have to deal with the disruption of their illness and the smell of their poverty. We don't want them hanging around the town square—and certainly not on a cross that we have to look at.

Fortunately, Dave and his mother outlived me. I left Way Station to pursue what I believed to be loftier goals. More mature staff succeeded me.

I returned several years later. Over the next ten years, we all grew older together—Dave, his mother, and I. Dave's rage dulled a bit with time, and his mother began to see us as difficult cousins—always making mistakes but at least committed. With a new baby of my own, I began to realize that the mother's anger was, in fact, fierce love. To better serve Dave and the most difficult clients like him, Way Station deepened its expertise and creativity. After Dave failed repeatedly in Way Station housing, and no local landlord would rent to him again, we brokered a creative solution, assisting his mother to purchase Dave a condo into which we provided staff support. When his mother's financial resources were exhausted, we worked with a reluctant bank that was assigned as his guardian by the VA, and we included the bank trustee as part of Dave's comprehensive care team.

Although Dave's memory was not good, he never seemed to forget his past relationship with me. When I returned to Way Station, and then almost every day for the years thereafter, Dave cursed me, convinced that I was embezzling his money. He needed Way Station desperately, but he wanted nothing to do with me.

It was the summer of 2000 when Way Station needed Dave.

We had started a small outpatient program in another county, and we were struggling to develop some needed housing. We were renting five units scattered among two apartment complexes, and problems were mounting. The landlords were trying to evict us because neighbors expressed concerns about our clients. We were losing a lot of money because of the inefficiency of staffing the scattered units. About to close the entire program in the county, we made one last-ditch effort.

We identified a perfect property—a small, home-like apartment building in an established neighborhood that would offer the residents the privacy and normalcy of single apartments. And yet, it would also provide the efficiency of centralized staffing and, most importantly, the potential for a Housing and Urban Development

(HUD) grant to purchase the property. The future of this program rested on our ability to convince the reluctant owners of the building, a middle-aged couple, to lease the property to us with an option to sell, should we secure the HUD grant. The owners were concerned about the impact of a mental health group home on the neighborhood and on their friends who still lived there. I tried to allay their fears, and I evaded their request to travel to Way Station's headquarters in the next county to see our programs there. I felt that even one small scene would sour the deal. But the owners insisted on coming before they would make a decision.

I elected to give the tour myself so I could hide the more difficult parts of our community—our more disabled clients. I artfully avoided the smoking area and eased the couple past Dave and a couple other clients who looked—or smelled—like the kind of person a neighborhood would not want.

We finally got up to my office relatively unscathed, but I knew we were losing them—I could see it in their eyes as they watched our clients shuffling around. They asked for a few minutes alone in my office to talk with each other, and I agreed.

When I came back five minutes later, my greatest fears were realized: Dave had wandered into my office and was talking to the couple! Braced for defeat, I raced in as Dave was leaving. But to my shock, the couple smiled and remarked how nice Dave was and that if he was the type of person who would be living in their apartment building, they would be proud to rent and sell it to us.

Evidently, Dave touched something deep within the wife's heart that reminded her of her mother who was suffering from Alzheimer's. Despite my efforts to hide it, the worst of Way Station burst in and became the best. When we needed him the most, Dave uncharacteristically held it together—and was downright charming—for five incredibly important minutes. Perhaps the only five minutes in his tortured life that he did shine. Maybe the only five minutes in his life that he was needed and permitted to shine.

We executed the lease, and Way Station was awarded the highly competitive HUD grant to purchase and renovate the apartment building. The grant included operational funding from HUD for forty years, and with that grant, we were able to expand the residential and outpatient programs, which now serve over 1,500 people every year.

Unlike other diseases, mental illness is often associated with fault and stigma, which dilute the compassion that the suffering individuals and their families deserve. I gave up on Dave because I blamed him for his aggressive behavior, his refusal to take medication, and his alcohol abuse, which compounded his mental illness.

And I blamed his mother for her pushiness and refusal to settle for lifetime institutionalization of her son. I blamed the couple who were cowering under the peer pressure of discrimination. And, at some level, I supposed I blamed myself for some or all of it, or I wouldn't have tried to hide Dave and the underbelly of Way Station from the couple when they visited.

Dave taught me that none of us was to blame for our various limitations that had brought us together; we were all called to keep our hearts open to God's power—even when we wanted so badly to give up.

Dave died of cancer several months after we purchased and occupied the building. He was finally taken down from his cross. But this time, thank God, it wasn't me trying to hide him.

FOURTEENTH STATION

Jesus Is Laid in the Tomb

Al Rose

When I think of Jesus suffering and dying, I think of so many people at Way Station who carry their invisible crosses with them everywhere they go. I think of Cal and Patrick and Shirley, the characters of previous stories. However, when I contemplate the fourteenth station, the burial of Jesus, I mostly think about Vinnie—or Vincente as he was baptized.

Tragically, there are people for whom the cross of depression cannot be alleviated. Vinnie was one, a young Latino who came from a very attentive family. Of small, wiry build, black-haired, with eyes so dark they looked black, he was a handsome fellow. But his greatest gifts were his quick intelligence and considerable breadth of knowledge. His parents had sought the best of help for him, beyond Way Station, that they

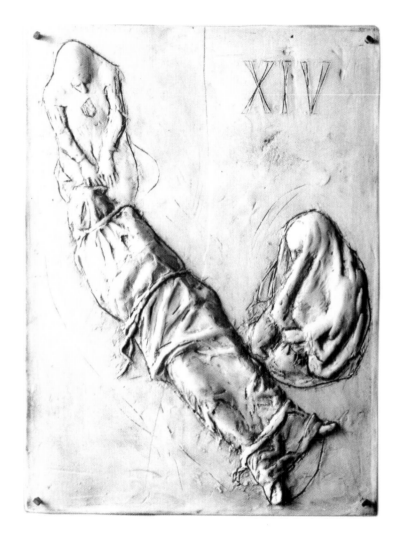

could afford on modest pensions, but to little avail. He struggled bravely, and when he was at relative peace, he was a stimulating student.

He always sat at the head of the table in the room where we met. If he was late, I jokingly reserved that seat for him, so that he could lead the discussions. That is where I saw him the most, at the head of that long table, five seats ranged down each side, and I at the end facing him. Everyone seemed quite willing to grant him that place.

He loved discussion, but found films less than stimulating and would complain when I was going to show one. He loved to talk and to dispute and to learn that way. However, in our group for men, he would deign to watch films about famous men, because there were yet things in those films that he did not know. But, of course, after the film, he plunged with gusto into discussion of the virtues and flaws of these men.

Although he had had to drop out of college because of depression, he had absorbed a great deal and had kept up by reading the newspapers avidly. He could tell us things about which he had a surprising fund of knowledge that none of us knew, and about politics that few of us had absorbed.

Speak about a president of the United States and Vinnie could explain the politics of the man's election. For instance, we learned that Abraham Lincoln was nominated by his advocates' having stacked the available spaces in the hall and then locking the doors. That led to a fierce and wonderful discussion about President Lincoln, a battle Vinnie clearly relished.

Speak about a president's private life and he could tell us that Mary Todd had lured Lincoln into marriage by seducing him. The next morning, Lincoln, the honorable man, felt he had to propose marriage, as she knew he would. We also learned that Lincoln had suffered with depression his entire life.

Vinnie told us about Franklin Roosevelt's private struggles with his disability. Polio had crippled him so that he could not walk. He was a handsome man, had been strong and athletic, with considerable ambition. At first depression had overcome him, but then he had learned to walk with large braces on both legs, a fact that had been fairly well concealed during his political career by his aides, who helped him walk, and by hiding his legs behind the podium.

Both those stories were followed with particularly great interest by others in the class. At the time, I simply missed the fact that probably both Vinnie's interest and his classmates' interest were due in part to the fact that he and many of them suffered from depression and that all were painfully conscious of their mental health disability.

I rarely saw Vinnie's depression, except when he

passed me distractedly in the halls, during the times when he was in too much pain to attend classes. He reached for every lifeline he could find. He tried acupuncture when we discussed it in a segment on China. He tried religion. He began to carry a Bible and once asked me some questions about it. He was using the King James Version, so I suggested to him that he might want to try the Revised Standard, as that was in a simpler language for a beginner and also acknowledged to be one of the most faithful translations of the originals. His response was to ask me, in what I can only describe as a plaintive way, if I thought Jesus would be angry with him if he didn't use Jesus's version. His concern may have stemmed from the fact that his introduction to the Bible had been by someone who believed it to be the only valid version. Or it could have been by the terror of scrupulosity suffered by some clients. I replied to him by urging him try the Revised Standard, adding that I didn't think Jesus would be angry. Vinnie's face was so pained. This was in the hall at the end of the class. People were passing between us, so there was no more conversation about the Bible, and we never went back to it. I have thought since about that brief encounter.

I hope that I did not take away from him what might have been his last effort to pull himself out of his excruciating depression, because not too long after that,

I was at Vinnie's funeral. He had checked into a hotel and had slit his wrists.

At the modest funeral parlor, small rooms and faded, stuffed furniture, where the funeral took place, I met his parents. They were kind and gentle people, with fairly strong Latin accents, obviously worn down by so many years of trying to find help for him, beyond Way Station. In doing so, they had exhausted the meager amount they had set aside for their own retirement. They were devastated by having lost the battle but seemed in a quiet way relieved that he was now out of his terrible struggle.

This sort of thing happens once in a while among people with mental illness and their families, a tragic consequence of the failure of available medicines and of many conscientious people simply being unable to alleviate the terrible pain of someone's depression. There was a small, perfunctory service at the parlor, presided over by a minister who had not known him. Later, there was a small luncheon at a modest, nearby café. Several staff and clients from Way Station joined his parents and me. That small band sat quietly around the table. We grieved for Vinnie with his parents. Some of us felt our own grief. Vinnie, with his intellectual energy and gusto for discussion, had brought sweet moments to our days.

The spiritual writer Michael Main has told the story

of his visit to Mother Teresa's hospice. At the end of the long room, lined on both sides with the dying, was a curtained area. Inside was the tub in which the sisters washed the emaciated bodies of those found by her and her staff on the streets of Calcutta, picked up and brought in to care for, to be given a dignified death by loving hands. Over the tub were the words "Body of Christ." So literal and so powerful and so convincing a reading of Jesus's question in Matthew 25: "Where were you when I was sick?"

I knew that I had been walking with the sick Vinnie.

And I had been walking with Jesus on the way of the cross.

And I had seen him into his tomb.

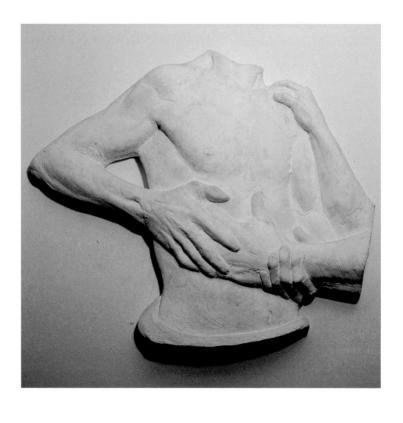

Jesus Rises from the Dead

Scott Rose

Several years after Melissa grieved the loss of her babies in the cemetery with Fred, she became pregnant yet again, but this time by another Way Station client, Charles, who was a wonderful man but felt unable to help raise the child because of his own severe mental illness. As a result, we moved toward adoption as the typical solution. With a recurring history of intense psychoses and suicide attempts, Melissa was in no position, much less state of mind, to raise a baby. The child welfare system did not have the expertise to deal with a mother with severe mental illness, and the adult mental health system had no resources or experience to care for babies. Worse yet, some of her psychotropic medications had to be discontinued because of the pregnancy.

Several staff members approached me to ask if I

would consider letting Melissa raise the baby in the group home. They had noticed to their surprise that Melissa's mental health was improving rather than deteriorating as the pregnancy continued. They hypothesized that the newfound purpose of having a baby, and the love it stimulated, were creating mental stability for Melissa. They said everyone was willing to pitch in to help, and they offered to contact and coordinate the numerous agencies that would need to be involved.

To this day, I'm not sure what caused me to say yes. It was my first year as CEO. I—and Way Station—had everything to lose. As an attorney, I knew all the liability risks to Way Station with a very ill, unmedicated mother and her newborn baby in one of our group homes. But in the end, it was a combination of Melissa's compelling request for redemption, the staff's inspiring commitment, and my recognition that the larger Way Station community needed some life and hope in the midst of recent tragedies related to other clients and an across-the-board burn-out of employees.

Several months later Jimmy was born. He was the resurrection of Melissa's lost babies. And a resurrection of lost lives and hope for the larger Way Station community.

Two weeks after Jimmy's birth, a large group of staff and clients gathered for a memorial service in the outpatient program building to grieve for three clients who had died prematurely. A sense of darkness and despair filled the room, as rain literally poured against the windows. Just as we were about to end, Melissa and Charles bounded in unexpectedly with the baby to introduce him for the first time to the Way Station community. People excitedly cleared the table of the torn photos of deceased clients and propped the car seat up in their place. The group surrounded the little family to tickle, coo, and giggle.

Jesus's resurrection unfolded before me. I realized that Melissa's tragedy-filled life triumphed over death, as did life for Way Station in general.

For the first three months after Jimmy's birth, Way Station staff volunteered to pull all-night shifts to support Melissa and the baby. I would sometimes wake up in the middle of the night in my own house in another section of town and would wonder how they were doing at the group home, and if they were awake nursing. I would imagine the baby nightlight shining in the dark, a small but sure beacon of new life and hope.

For several decades I have cherished that image of resurrection at Way Station. It has given me hope whenever I desperately needed it. But it is important to recognize that God—and that nightlight—did not eliminate this family's darkness, and that the reality of resurrection in mental health recovery is not diminished, even though it often is followed by failure and death yet again. The hope of recovery is that all of those who are impacted by the illness—those suffering with it, their families, and their caregivers—will achieve net progress and insight over time in spite of the inevitable setbacks and, sometimes, tragedies. As Therese noted in the Prologue, the goal is often to help people, including families and caregivers, *manage* the symptoms, rather than to eliminate them—in the same way that light can help us manage darkness as opposed to dispelling it. In the journey of recovery with mental illness, our faith will wither and die if our spirituality is contingent upon the hope that if we can get through the first fourteen stations of the cross, our pain will be resolved or dramatically reduced when we get to the last one. In contrast, a more enduring spiritual perspective is that reliving with Jesus his suffering reminds us that we are not alone in ours, that there can be purpose in our pain, and that we will periodically experience redemption and renewal that will be *good enough* to keep us going—even if we have to walk through the stations again.

Melissa died of natural causes two years after Jimmy was born. Evidence of his own resurrection, Charles stepped up and took responsibility for raising Jimmy. And he did it wonderfully. Most importantly, Charles talked often about his mental illness with his son, emphasizing the importance of taking his psychiatric medicine, teaching the boy how to manage—not prevent—

mental illness. But then, tragedy and darkness struck again: Charles also died of natural causes, leaving Jimmy an orphan at age eleven, with the daze of pain and struggle gathering in his freckled eyes. Charles's saintly parents are now raising Jimmy.

For Jimmy and his family, while their experiences of resurrection did not stop their suffering, it did provide them hope needed to continue the journey. Both parents found personal redemption through their love for their son. Jimmy had his mother for two years, and the knowledge for the rest of his life that she loved him so much that she battled through the terror of mental illness in order that she could bear and nurse him. And his father taught him the most valuable lesson of his life: how to manage challenge, fear, and pain.

The family who walked in darkness—and the Way Station community who walked with them—saw a great light.

ABOUT THE AUTHORS
AND ARTIST

Scott Rose is CEO and General Counsel of Way Station, Inc., a nonprofit community mental health organization that serves over three thousand low-income adults and children in four Maryland counties. He has worked at Way Station for thirty years, serving in various other positions, including van driver, direct-service counselor, administrator, and attorney. His writing reflects his own personal views, not those of Way Station, which is a nonsectarian organization.

Fred Wenner was a pastor in the United Church of Christ for forty years, during which time he and his wife parented fifty-three foster children, many of whom had emotional challenges. They adopted four, adding them to their family of four biological children. Three of the four children about whom he writes received mental health services from Way Station. Fred views his parish ministry and his community leadership in peace and justice as having been informed by the contemplative spirituality of the Roman Catholic tradition. Directly experiencing major depression caused by Lyme Disease, Fred does outreach ministry to people with mental illness in addition to active participation in his church community.

Al Rose was as a university professor of literature for thirty-one years, publishing professionally on nineteenth-century Jesuit poet Gerard Manley Hopkins. He was involved in campus ministry and served as lay Catholic chaplain in the county jail. He retired early, answering a call to ordination in the permanent diaconate of the Roman Catholic Church and subsequently worked as a chaplain at the Maryland State Penitentiary's Maximum Security Prison. Later he became chaplain at an inner-city hospice. On retirement, he served as a volunteer for a program affiliated with Way Station.

Therese Borchard is the founder and executive director of Beyond Blue Foundation and the host of ProjectBeyondBlue.com, an online community for people living with chronic depression and other mood disorders. She writes the blog Sanity Break for Everyday Health and is associate editor at PsychCentral.com. Therese is the author of *Beyond Blue: Surviving Depression & Anxiety and*

Making the Most of Bad Genes, The Pocket Therapist: An Emotional Survival Kit, and is coeditor, with Michael Leach, of the national bestseller, *I Like Being Catholic: Treasured Traditions, Rituals, and Stories.* She speaks throughout the country on the topic of faith and mental illness, and can be found at thereseborchard.com.

Homer Yost is a professional sculptor who is a former Way Station client with bipolar disorder. The artwork in this book comes from a series of relief sculptures, "The Stations of the Cross," which were commissioned by a Roman Catholic parish. Homer has been sculpting and drawing for more than thirty-five years. He received his MFA in sculpture and drawing from the University of North Carolina at Greensboro in 1984. He has exhibited his work in galleries around the country as well as in England and Italy.